Underground Clinical Vignettes

Vignettes

Internal Medicine II

Underground
Clinical Vignettes
Internal Medicine II

FOURTH EDITION

Sandra I. Kim, M.D., Ph.D.
Resident in Internal Medicine
Beth Israel Deaconess Medical Center
Harvard Medical School
Boston, Massachusetts

Todd A. Swanson, M.D., Ph.D.
Resident in Radiation Oncology
William Beaumont Hospital
Royal Oak, Michigan

Wolters Kluwer | Lippincott Williams & Wilkins
Health
Philadelphia • Baltimore • New York • London
Buenos Aires • Hong Kong • Sydney • Tokyo

Acquisitions editor: Nancy Anastasi Duffy
Developmental editor: Nancy Hoffmann
Managing editor: Kelly Horvath
Production editor: Kevin Johnson
Marketing manager: Jennifer Kuklinski
Designer: Doug Smock
Compositor: International Typesetting and Composition

WB 18

A080338

© 2007 by Lippincott Williams & Wilkins
UCV Step 2 *Internal Medicine II*, Fourth Edition

Lippincott Williams & Wilkins, a Wolters Kluwer business.

351 West Camden Street   530 Walnut Street
Baltimore, MD 21201   Philadelphia, PA 19106

9 8 7 6 5 4 3 2 1

Library of Congress Cataloging-in-Publication Data

Kim, Sandra.
    Internal medicine II.—4th ed. / Sandra I. Kim, Todd A. Swanson.
        p. ; cm.—(Underground clinical vignettes. Step 2)
    Includes index.
    Rev. ed. of: Internal medicine / Vikhas Bhushan . . . [et al.]. 3rd ed. c2005.
    ISBN 0-7817-6836-5
    1. Internal medicine—Case studies.   2. Physicians—Licenses—United States—Examinations—Study guides.   I. Title.   II. Title: Internal medicine 2.   III. Title: Internal medicine two.   IV. Series.
    [DNLM: 1. Internal Medicine—Problems and Exercises.   WB 18.2 K49i 2007]
    RC66.I5762 2007
    616—dc22

                                                                                        2007036696

DISCLAIMER
    Care has been taken to confirm the accuracy of the information present and to describe generally accepted practices. However, the authors, editors, and publisher are not responsible for errors or omissions or for any consequences from application of the information in this book and make no warranty, expressed or implied, with respect to the currency, completeness, or accuracy of the contents of the publication. Application of this information in a particular situation remains the professional responsibility of the prac-titioner; the clinical treatments described and recommended may not be considered absolute and universal recommendations.
    The authors, editors, and publisher have exerted every effort to ensure that drug selection and dosage set forth in this text are in accordance with the current recommendations and practice at the time of publica-tion. However, in view of ongoing research, changes in government regulations, and the constant flow of information relating to drug therapy and drug reactions, the reader is urged to check the package insert for each drug for any change in indications and dosage and for added warnings and precautions. This is par-ticularly important when the recommended agent is a new or infrequently employed drug.
    Some drugs and medical devices presented in this publication have Food and Drug Administration (FDA) clearance for limited use in restricted research settings. It is the responsibility of the health care provider to ascertain the FDA status of each drug or device planned for use in their clinical practice.

To purchase additional copies of this book, call our customer service department at **(800) 638-3030** or fax orders to **(301) 223-2320**. International customers should call **(301) 223-2300**.

Visit Lippincott Williams & Wilkins on the Internet: http://www.lww.com. Lippincott Williams & Wilkins cus-tomer service representatives are available from 8:30 am to 6:00 pm, EST.

dedications

Dedicated to the patients we care for.

preface

First published in 1999, the Underground Clinical Vignettes (UCV) series has provided thousands of students with a highly effective review tool as they prepare for medical examinations, particularly the USMLE Step 1 and 2 examinations. Designed as a quick study guide, each UCV book contains patient-centered clinical cases that highlight a range of medical diagnoses.

With this new edition of Step 2 UCV, we have incorporated feedback from medical students across the country to provide updated cases with expanded treatment and discussion sections. Every title has more cases, drawing from a broader area within each discipline. A new two-page format enables readers to formulate an initial diagnosis prior to reading the "answer" to each case. The inclusion of relevant magnetic resonance images, x-rays, and photographs allows students to more readily visualize the physical presentation of each case. Breakout boxes, tables, and algorithms have been added, along with 20 all-new, board-format questions-and-answers, making this edition of UCV an ideal source of information for examination review, classroom discussion, and clinical rotations.

The clinical vignettes in this Step 2 series have been revised and updated to reflect current medical thinking on medication, pathogenesis, epidemiology, management, and complications. Although each case presents most of the signs, symptoms, and diagnostic findings for a particular illness, patients typically do not present with such a "complete" picture either clinically or on a medical examination. Cases are not meant to simulate a potential real patient or an examination vignette.

Access to Lippincott Williams & Wilkins (LWW)'s online companion site, ThePoint, will be offered as a premium with the purchase of the UCV Step 2 bundle. Benefits include an online test link and 160 additional new board-format questions covering all UCV subject areas.

We hope you will find the UCV series informative and useful. We welcome any feedback, suggestions, or corrections you have about this series. Please contact us at LWW.com/medstudent.

contributors

Series Editors

Sandra I. Kim, M.D., Ph.D.
Resident in Internal Medicine
Beth Israel Deaconess Medical Center
Harvard Medical School
Boston, Massachusetts

Todd A. Swanson, M.D., Ph.D.
Resident in Radiation Oncology
William Beaumont Hospital
Royal Oak, Michigan

Contributing Editors

Suzelle Luc, M.D., M.P.H.
Resident in Internal Medicine
Beth Israel Deaconess Medical Center
Harvard Medical School
Boston, Massachusetts

Anita Vanka, M.D.
Resident in Internal Medicine
Beth Israel Deaconess Medical Center
Harvard Medical School
Boston, Massachusetts

Internal Medicine II—Contributors

Eyal Oren, M.D., Ph.D.
Yung Chyung, M.D.
Aleena Suryadevara Banerji, M.D.
Nisha Basu, M.D.

acknowledgments

Our great thanks to the housestaff and faculty from Beth Israel Deaconess, Massachusetts General, Brigham and Women's, and Children's Hospitals in Boston, whose clinical cases, revisions, and suggestions were indispensable to this series. Thanks to the editors at Lippincott Williams & Wilkins, especially Nancy Hoffmann, who worked overtime on these books.

abbreviations

A-a	alveolar-arterial (oxygen gradient)	ATN	acute tubular necrosis
AAA	abdominal aortic aneurysm	ATPase	adenosine triphosphatase
ABCs	airway, breathing, circulation	ATRA	all-*trans*-retinoic acid
ABGs	arterial blood gases	AV	arteriovenous, atrioventricular
ABPA	allergic bronchopulmonary aspergillosis	AVPD	avoidant personality disorder
		AXR	abdominal x-ray
ABVD	adriamycin, bleomycin, vinblastine, dacarbazine (chemotherapy)	AZT	azidothymidine (zidovudine)
		BCG	bacille Calmette-Guérin
ACE	angiotensin-converting enzyme	BE	barium enema
ACTH	adrenocorticotropic hormone	BP	blood pressure
ADA	adenosine deaminase, American Diabetic Association	BPD	borderline personality disorder
		BPH	benign prostatic hypertrophy
ADH	antidiuretic hormone	BPK	B-cell progenitor kinase
ADHD	attention-deficit hyperactivity disorder	BPM	beats per minute
		BUN	blood urea nitrogen
AED	automatic external defibrillator	CAA	cerebral amyloid angiopathy
AFP	α-fetoprotein	CABG	coronary artery bypass grafting
AI	aortic insufficiency	CAD	coronary artery disease
AICD	automatic internal cardiac defibrillator	CALLA	common acute lymphoblastic leukemia antigen
AIDS	acquired immunodeficiency syndrome	C-ANCA	cytoplasmic antineutrophil cytoplasmic antibody
ALL	acute lymphocytic leukemia	CAO	chronic airway obstruction
ALS	amyotrophic lateral sclerosis	CAP	community-acquired pneumonia
ALT	alanine aminotransferase	CBC	complete blood count
AML	acute myelogenous leukemia	CBD	common bile duct
AMP	adenosine monophosphate	CBT	cognitive behavioral therapy
ANA	antinuclear antibody	CCU	cardiac care unit
ANCA	antineutrophil cytoplasmic antibody	CD	cluster of differentiation
		CDC	Centers for Disease Control
Angio	angiography	CEA	carcinoembryonic antigen
AP	anteroposterior	CF	cystic fibrosis
aPTT	activated partial thromboplastin time	CFTR	cystic fibrosis transmembrane regulator
ARDS	adult respiratory distress syndrome	CFU	colony-forming unit
ARF	acute renal failure	CHF	congestive heart failure
AS	ankylosing spondylitis	CJD	Creutzfeldt–Jakob disease
ASA	acetylsalicylic acid	CK	creatine kinase
5-ASA	5-aminosalicylic acid	CK-MB	creatine kinase, MB fraction
ASD	atrial septal defect	CLL	chronic lymphocytic leukemia
ASO	antistreptolysin O	CML	chronic myelogenous leukemia
AST	aspartate aminotransferase	CMV	cytomegalovirus
ATLS	Advanced Trauma Life Support (protocol)	CN	cranial nerve
		CNS	central nervous system

CO	cardiac output
COPD	chronic obstructive pulmonary disease
CPAP	continuous positive airway pressure
CPK	creatine phosphokinase
CPR	cardiopulmonary resuscitation
CRP	C-reactive protein
CSF	cerebrospinal fluid
CT	computed tomography
CVA	cerebrovascular accident
CXR	chest x-ray
D&C	dilatation and curettage
DAF	decay-accelerating factor
DC	direct current
DEXA	dual-energy x-ray absorptiometry
DHEA	dehydroepiandrosterone
DIC	disseminated intravascular coagulation
DIP	distal interphalangeal (joint)
DKA	diabetic ketoacidosis
DL_{CO}	diffusing capacity of carbon monoxide
DM	diabetes mellitus
DMD	Duchenne's muscular dystrophy
DNA	deoxyribonucleic acid
DNase	deoxyribonuclease
dsDNA	double-stranded DNA
DTP	diphtheria, tetanus, pertussis (vaccine)
DTRs	deep tendon reflexes
DTs	delirium tremens
DUB	dysfunctional uterine bleeding
DVT	deep venous thrombosis
EBV	Epstein–Barr virus
ECG	electrocardiography
Echo	echocardiography
ECMO	extracorporeal membrane oxygenation
EDTA	ethylenediamine tetraacetic acid
EEG	electroencephalography
EF	ejection fraction
EGD	esophagogastroduodenoscopy
E:I	expiratory-to-inspiratory (ratio)
ELISA	enzyme-linked immunosorbent assay
EM	electron microscopy
EMG	electromyography
ER	emergency room

ERCP	endoscopic retrograde cholangiopancreatography
ESR	erythrocyte sedimentation rate
EtOH	ethanol
FDA	Food and Drug Administration
Fe_{Na}	fractional excretion of sodium
FEV_1	forced expiratory volume in 1 second
FIGO	International Federation of Gynecology and Obstetrics (classification)
FIO_2	fraction of inspired oxygen
FNA	fine-needle aspiration
FRC	functional residual capacity
FSH	follicle-stimulating hormone
FTA	fluorescent treponemal antibody
FTA-ABS	fluorescent treponemal antibody absorption test
5-FU	5-fluorouracil
FVC	forced vital capacity
G6PD	glucose-6-phosphate dehydrogenase
GA	gestational age
GABA	gamma-aminobutyric acid
GABHS	group A β-hemolytic streptococcus
GAD	generalized anxiety disorder
GBM	glomerular basement membrane
G-CSF	granulocyte colony-stimulating factor
GERD	gastroesophageal reflux disease
GFR	glomerular filtration rate
GGT	gamma-glutamyltransferase
GI	gastrointestinal
GnRH	gonadotropin-releasing hormone
GU	genitourinary
HAV	hepatitis A virus
Hb	hemoglobin
HBcAg	hepatitis B core antigen
HBsAg	hepatitis B surface antigen
HBV	hepatitis B virus
hCG	human chorionic gonadotropin
HCl	hydrogen chloride
HCO_3	bicarbonate
Hct	hematocrit
HCV	hepatitis C virus
HDL	high-density lipoprotein
HEENT	head, eyes, ears, nose, and throat
HELLP	hemolysis, elevated liver enzymes, low platelets (syndrome)

HEV	hepatitis E virus	LAMB	lentigines, atrial myxoma, blue nevi (syndrome)
HGPRT	hypoxanthine-guanine phosphoribosyltransferase	LD	Leishman-Donovan (body)
HHV	human herpesvirus	LDH	lactate dehydrogenase
5-HIAA	5-hydroxyindoleacetic acid	LDL	low-density lipoprotein
HIDA	hepato-iminodiacetic acid (scan)	LES	lower esophageal sphincter
		LFTs	liver function tests
HIV	human immunodeficiency virus	LH	luteinizing hormone
HLA	human leukocyte antigen	LHRH	luteinizing hormone–releasing hormone
HPF	high-power field		
HPI	history of present illness	LKM	liver-kidney microsomal (antibody)
HPV	human papillomavirus	LMN	lower motor neuron
HR	heart rate	LP	lumbar puncture
HRCT	high-resolution computed tomography	L/S	lecithin-to-sphingomyelin (ratio)
		LSD	lysergic acid diethylamide
HS	hereditary spherocytosis	LV	left ventricle, left ventricular
HSG	hysterosalpingography	LVH	left ventricular hypertrophy
HSV	herpes simplex virus	Lytes	electrolytes
HUS	hemolytic-uremic syndrome	Mammo	mammography
IABC	intra-aortic balloon counter-pulsation	MAO	monoamine oxidase (inhibitor)
		MAP	mean arterial pressure
ICA	internal carotid artery	MCA	middle cerebral artery
ICD	implantable cardiac defibrillator	MCHC	mean corpuscular hemoglobin concentration
ICP	intracranial pressure		
ICU	intensive care unit	MCP	metacarpophalangeal (joint)
ID/CC	identification and chief complaint	MCV	mean corpuscular volume
IDDM	insulin-dependent diabetes mellitus	MDMA	3,4-methylene-dioxymetham-phetamine ("Ecstasy")
IE	infectious endocarditis	MEN	multiple endocrine neoplasia
IFA	immunofluorescent antibody	MGUS	monoclonal gammopathy of undetermined origin
Ig	immunoglobulin		
IL	interleukin	MHC	major histocompatibility complex
IM	infectious mononucleosis, intramuscular	MI	myocardial infarction
		MIBG	metaiodobenzylguanidine
INH	isoniazid	MMR	measles, mumps, rubella (vaccine)
INR	International Normalized Ratio		
123-ISS	iodine-123-labeled somatostatin	MPTP	1-methyl-4-phenyl-tetrahy-dropyridine
IUD	intrauterine device		
IUGR	intrauterine growth retardation	MR	magnetic resonance (imaging)
IV	intravenous	mRNA	messenger ribonucleic acid
IVC	inferior vena cava	MRSA	methicillin-resistant *Staphylococcus* aureus
IVIG	intravenous immunoglobulin		
IVP	intravenous pyelography	MS	multiple sclerosis
JRA	juvenile rheumatoid arthritis	MTP	metatarsophalangeal (joint)
JVD	jugular venous distention	MuSK	muscle-specific kinase
JVP	jugular venous pressure	MVA	motor vehicle accident
KOH	potassium hydroxide	NADPH	reduced nicotinamide adenine dinucleotide phosphate
KS	Kaposi's sarcoma		
KUB	kidney, ureter, bladder	NAME	nevi, atrial myxoma, myxoid neu-rofibroma, ephelides (syndrome)
LA	left atrium		

NG	nasogastric		RBC	red blood cell
NIDDM	non-insulin-dependent diabetes mellitus		RDW	red-cell distribution width
NMDA	*N*-methyl-D-aspartate		REM	rapid eye movement
NPO	nil per os (nothing by mouth)		RF	rheumatoid factor
NSAID	nonsteroidal anti-inflammatory drug		RhoGAM	Rh immune globulin
Nuc	nuclear medicine		RNA	ribonucleic acid
OCD	obsessive-compulsive disorder		RPR	rapid plasma reagin
OCP	oral contraceptive pill		RR	respiratory rate
OCPD	obsessive-compulsive personality disorder		RS	Reed-Sternberg (cell)
17-OHP	17-hydroxyprogesterone		RSV	respiratory syncytial virus
OPC	organophosphate and carbamate		RTA	renal tubular acidosis
OS	opening snap		RUQ	right upper quadrant
OTC	over the counter		RV	residual volume, right ventricle, right ventricular
PA	posteroanterior		RVH	right ventricular hypertrophy
2-PAM	pralidoxime		SA	sinoatrial
P-ANCA	perinuclear antineutrophil cytoplasmic antibody		SAH	subarachnoid hemorrhage
Pao_2	partial pressure of oxygen		Sao_2	oxygen saturation in arterial blood
PAS	periodic acid Schiff		SBE	subacute bacterial endocarditis
PBS	peripheral blood smear		SBFT	small bowel follow-through
Pco_2	partial pressure of carbon dioxide		SC	subcutaneous
PCOD	polycystic ovary disease		SCC	squamous cell carcinoma
PCP	phencyclidine		SIADH	syndrome of inappropriate secretion of antidiuretic hormone
PCR	polymerase chain reaction		SIDS	sudden infant death syndrome
PCV	polycythemia vera		SLE	systemic lupus erythematosus
PDA	patent ductus arteriosus		SMA	smooth muscle antibody
PE	physical exam		SSPE	subacute sclerosing panencephalitis
PEEP	positive end-expiratory pressure		SSRI	selective serotonin reuptake inhibitor
PET	positron emission tomography		STD	sexually transmitted disease
PFTs	pulmonary function tests		SZPD	schizoid personality disorder
PID	pelvic inflammatory disease		T_3	triiodothyronine
PIP	proximal interphalangeal (joint)		T_4	thyroxine
PKU	phenylketonuria		TAB	therapeutic abortion
PMI	point of maximal impulse		TB	tuberculosis
PMN	polymorphonuclear (leukocyte)		TBSA	total body surface area
PO	per os (by mouth)		TCA	tricyclic antidepressant
Po_2	partial pressure of oxygen		TCD	transcranial Doppler
PPD	purified protein derivative		TD	tardive dyskinesia
PROM	premature rupture of membranes		TENS	transcutaneous electrical nerve stimulation
PRPP	phosphoribosyl pyrophosphate		TFTs	thyroid function tests
PSA	prostate-specific antigen		THC	*trans*-tetrahydrocannabinol
PT	prothrombin time		TIA	transient ischemic attack
PTE	pulmonary thromboembolism		TIBC	total iron-binding capacity
PTH	parathyroid hormone		TIPS	transjugular intrahepatic portosystemic shunt
PTSD	post-traumatic stress disorder			
PTT	partial thromboplastin time			
RA	rheumatoid arthritis, right atrial			

TLC	total lung capacity	US	ultrasound
TMJ	temporomandibular joint (syndrome)	UTI	urinary tract infection
		UV	ultraviolet
TMP-SMX	trimethoprim-sulfamethoxazole	VCUG	voiding cystourethrogram
TNF	tumor necrosis factor	VDRL	Venereal Disease Research Laboratory
TNM	tumor, node, metastasis (staging)		
ToRCH	*Toxoplasma,* rubella, CMV, herpes zoster	VF	ventricular fibrillation
		VIN	vulvar intraepithelial neoplasia
tPA	tissue plasminogen activator	VLDL	very low density lipoprotein
TPO	thyroid peroxidase	VMA	vanillylmandelic acid
TRAP	tartrate-resistant acid phosphatase	V/Q	ventilation-perfusion (ratio)
TRH	thyrotropin-releasing hormone	VS	vital signs
TSH	thyroid-stimulating hormone	VSD	ventricular septal defect
TSS	toxic shock syndrome	VT	ventricular tachycardia
TSST	toxic shock syndrome toxin	vWF	von Willebrand factor
TTP	thrombotic thrombocytopenic purpura	VZIG	varicella-zoster immune globulin
TUBD	transurethral balloon dilatation	VZV	varicella-zoster virus
TUIP	transurethral incision of the prostate	WAGR	Wilms' tumor, aniridia, ambiguous genitalia, mental retardation (syndrome)
TURP	transurethral resection of the prostate		
		WBC	white blood cell
UA	urinalysis	WG	Wegener's granulomatosis
UGI	upper GI (series)	WPW	Wolff–Parkinson–White (syndrome)
UMN	upper motor neuron		
URI	upper respiratory infection	XR	x-ray

Underground Clinical Vignettes

Internal Medicine II

FOURTH EDITION

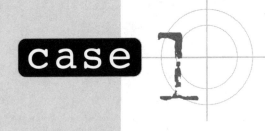

case 1

ID/CC A **37-year-old man** presents to his primary care physician with a history of **runny nose** and **sneezing.**

HPI Since childhood, he has had symptoms of rhinorrhea, sneezing, nasal congestion, and **nasal itching.** Occasionally, he has postnasal drip and throat clearing. He also complains of **itchy, watery eyes.** His symptoms occur year-round but are typically **worse in the spring.**

PE VS: normal. PE: conjunctival erythema; bilateral inferior turbinate swelling and pale swollen nasal mucosa but without polyps or bleeding, clear nasal discharge present bilaterally, no sinus tenderness; posterior pharynx with mucosal cobblestoning.

Labs CBC: eosinophils elevated.

Imaging None.

case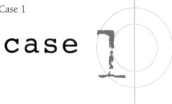

Allergic Rhinitis

Pathogenesis

Allergic rhinitis is triggered by **IgE-mediated responses to allergens.** On entering the nasal passage, allergens bind to allergen-specific IgE that is bound on the surface of mast cells. **Cross-linking of IgE activates mast cells,** which in turn leads to the release of a variety of mediators, such as **histamine, tryptase, kinins, prostaglandins, and leukotrienes.** These released mediators interact with other cells in the nasal mucosa, which leads to increased vascular permeability, vasodilation, and mucus production. Moreover, these mediators can activate nerve signaling within the nasal mucosa, resulting in the sensation of **itching** as well as sometimes triggering sneezing.

Epidemiology

20% of the population has allergic rhinitis. Individuals with a family history of atopy (such as allergic rhinitis, asthma, or eczema) have a significantly increased risk of developing allergic rhinitis. Tree pollen levels predominate in the spring, grass pollens in the summer, and weed pollens in autumn. Dust mites and molds are present year-round.

Management

Nasal corticosteroid sprays are very effective in treating nasal congestion as well as nasal itching, sneezing, and rhinorrhea and therefore are the cornerstone of management. **H1-receptor blockers** treat the symptoms of nasal itching, sneezing, and rhinorrhea and can be used as an adjunct. Skin testing can be performed by an allergist to identify the specific environmental allergens, followed by environmental control measures and immunotherapy, which can lead to decreased sensitivity to those allergens.

Complications

Allergic rhinitis results in 3.5 million lost workdays and 2 million missed school days each year.

Breakout Point

- Pale boggy turbinates with edema
- Nasal corticosteroids are the cornerstone of treatment
- Immunotherapy is effective in 70% to 80% of patients

■ TABLE 1-1 PHARMACOLOGIC OPTIONS FOR RHINITIS: EFFECTS ON SYMPTOMS

Agent	Sneezing	Itching	Congestion	Rhinorrhea	Eye Symptoms
Oral antihistamines	++	++	+/−	++	++
Nasal antihistamines	+	+	+	+	−
Intranasal corticosteroids	++	++	+++	++	+
Leukotriene modifiers	+	+	+	+	+
Oral decongestants	−	−	++	−	−
Nasal decongestants	−	−	+++	−	−
Nasal mast cell stabilizers	+	+	+	+	−
Topical anticholinergics	−	−	−	+++	−

+++, marked benefit; ++, substantial benefit; +, some benefit; +/−, minimal benefit; −, no benefit.

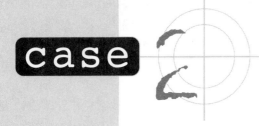

ID/CC A **56-year-old African-American man** with hypertension presents with **lip and tongue swelling** that started three days ago.

HPI He describes intermittent episodes of lip and tongue swelling that are **not associated with pruritus.** The episodes have lasted 24 hours in the past and resolved spontaneously. He denies any associated hives, chest tightness, or wheezing. He notes occasional dysphagia. He cannot associate any specific foods with these episodes. His only new medication is **lisinopril** that he began using 1 week ago to treat his hypertension.

PE VS: normal. PE: lip and tongue swelling, no uvular edema; no stridor heard on auscultation of the neck; lungs clear; skin with no rashes, no erythema.

Labs C4: 22 mg/dL (normal). C1 inhibitor level: 29 mg/dL (normal).

Imaging Laryngoscopy reveals glottic edema.

case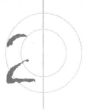

Angioedema

Pathogenesis

Angioedema is a **life-threatening event** associated with ACE inhibitor therapy. Many studies suggest that elevated bradykinin levels are responsible for ACE inhibitor angioedema, but the precise mechanism remains poorly understood. ACE inhibitor angioedema typically involves the mouth, lips, tongue, larynx, pharynx, and subglottic tissues. **Urticaria is absent.**

Epidemiology

Due to the large number of patients treated with this class of medications, **ACE inhibitors are the most frequent cause of angioedema seen in hospitals and emergency rooms.** Angioedema occurs in 0.1% to 0.7% of patients treated with ACE inhibitors with a 4- to 5-fold higher risk in African Americans. Approximately 1 in 3000 patients develops angioedema during the first week of treatment with ACE inhibitors. However, it is important to remember that ACE inhibitor related angioedema can occur several years after initiation of therapy.

Management

The treatment of angioedema depends on the severity of symptoms. If the airway is compromised, a patient may need to be intubated for airway protection. The patient should be admitted for observation until angioedema has completely resolved. Patients should be warned that they **can experience angioedema up to 2 weeks after discontinuation of the ACE inhibitor.** These patients should never use an ACE inhibitor again. Antihistamines, steroids, and epinephrine can be used, but they may not provide significant benefit.

Complications

Death can occur but it is very rare. With discontinuation of the ACE inhibitor, most patients recover without long-term sequelae.

Breakout Point

- Lip and tongue swelling
- Can occur years after starting ACE inhibitor.

■ TABLE 2-1 CAUSES OF ANGIOEDEMA

ACE inhibitors (20%–58%)
IgE-mediated allergic reaction to a food, drug, or environmental trigger (17%–33%)
C1 esterase inhibitor deficiency, either hereditary or acquired (<1%–2%)
NSAIDs
Chemical histamine release
Idiopathic causes (21%–59%)

case 3

ID/CC A **36-year-old woman** presents to the ER with **wheezing** and **shortness of breath** after taking aspirin earlier in the day.

HPI The patient has a **history of asthma,** chronic nasal congestion, and **nasal polyps.** She has a history of multiple polyp removal surgeries and has developed anosmia (loss of olfaction) over the years. Over the past year, she has noticed that **on days that she takes aspirin or ibuprofen, her asthma symptoms are more severe.** She reports that she does not develop any associated rash; itching; or swelling of her face, eyes, lips, tongue, or body. Today, after ingesting several doses of aspirin for her migraine, she developed wheezing and shortness of breath.

PE VS: normal. PE: inferior nasal turbinate swelling bilaterally with polyps visible; lungs with few scattered end-expiratory wheezes; skin with no rash or angioedema.

Labs None.

Imaging Rhinoscopy: large nasal polyp.

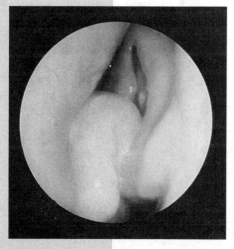

Figure 3-1. Rhinoscopy showing a large nasal polyp.

case 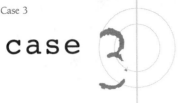3

Aspirin-sensitive Asthma

Pathogenesis

The triad of **asthma, nasal polyps, and aspirin sensitivity** is known as **"Samter's Triad"** and was first described in 1968. The enzyme cyclooxygenase-1 (COX-1) catalyzes the conversion of arachidonic acid to prostaglandins and thromboxanes. Aspirin and NSAIDs, however, inhibit COX-1, which leads to the excessive accumulation of arachidonic acid. Because arachidonic acid also is converted by the enzyme 5-lipoxygenase to form leukotrienes, the conversion of excess arachidonic acid leads to increased production of leukotrienes. Leukotrienes cause bronchoconstriction, mucus production, and eosinophil recruitment, which all exacerbate the asthma disease process.

Epidemiology

It has been estimated that as many as 20% of patients with asthma have aspirin-sensitivity.

Management

Aspirin and NSAIDs should be avoided. Acetaminophen is generally tolerated by aspirin-sensitive patients, but acetaminophen can inhibit COX-1 at high doses, and so **>1000 mg of acetaminophen should be avoided. Leukotriene receptor blockers** (such as montelukast) and **leukotriene synthesis inhibitors** (such as zileuton) are often effective in treating the asthma and nasal symptoms in aspirin-sensitive patients. Patients can be **desensitized** to aspirin and NSAIDs for specific conditions by an allergist under careful observation.

Complications

ASH-sensitive patients are at risk of developing recurrent nasal polyps.

Breakout Point

> Samter's Triad: Asthma, nasal polyps, aspirin sensitivity

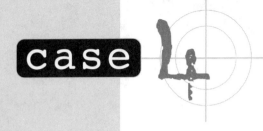

case

ID/CC A **35-year-old** man presents to his primary care physician with a 4-month history of **hives.**

HPI The patient complains of hives on a daily basis for the past 4 months. The hives can occur anywhere on his body and have led to significant **pruritus** and impairment of his daily activities. On days that his hives are especially severe, he has had **swelling of his lips and eyelids.** He has not noticed any correlation of his hives with any particular foods, medications, or other exposures.

PE VS: normal. PE: skin with numerous scattered raised, erythematous lesions of 10–15 mm diameter that blanch with pressure on the arms, legs, neck, chest, and abdomen.

Labs None.

Imaging None.

case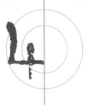

Chronic Urticaria

Pathogenesis

Urticaria is caused by the **activation of mast cells**, which release a variety of mediators, such as **histamine, tryptase, kinins, heparins, prostaglandins, and leukotrienes**. These released mediators lead to the formation of **wheals and erythema**. Chronic urticaria is defined as **urticaria lasting 6 weeks or longer** in duration. In contrast to acute urticaria, an allergic trigger is rarely identified. Causes of chronic urticaria that have been described include **autoimmune disease, thyroid disease, hepatitis virus infection, and physical stimuli** (such as heat, cold, sweat, contact, sunlight, or water). In many patients with idiopathic chronic urticaria, the causative factor may be an autoantibody to the high-affinity IgE receptor, which leads to triggering of the IgE receptor signaling pathway and activation of mast cells.

Epidemiology

Between 15% and 25% of the general population will develop urticaria at some point in their lives. Chronic urticaria, however, is considerably less common, and it has been estimated to occur in 0.1% to 0.5% of the population. A history of atopy is not associated with an increased risk of developing chronic urticaria.

Management

H1-receptor blockers are the mainstay of treatment of urticaria. Approximately 10%–15% of the histamine receptors in the skin are estimated to be H2 receptors, and so **adding an H2-receptor blocker** to an H1-receptor blocker may provide added relief. Unlike first-generation antihistamine medications (such as diphenhydramine), second-generation antihistamine medications (such as fexofenadine, loratadine, cetirizine) are generally much less sedating.

Complications

Chronic urticaria is generally not life-threatening, but can be debilitating due to severe itching. Most cases resolve within a year.

Breakout Point

- Chronic, >6 weeks
- Treat with antihistamines
- Usually benign

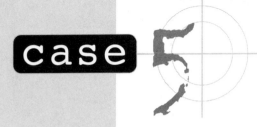

ID/CC A **42-year-old white woman** presents to the ER with **generalized hives, wheezing,** and a **feeling that she is about to pass out.**

HPI She was in her garden tending to her flowers an hour earlier when she was **stung by an insect.** Within **15 minutes,** she developed **flushing** followed by **itch and hives** throughout her body. She then began feeling her **throat tighten with difficulty breathing.** She felt some abdominal discomfort and nausea.

PE VS: afebrile, tachycardia (HR 120), hypotension (BP 90/50). PE: tremulous, diaphoretic, with audible wheeze; tearing and rhinorrhea with flushing of the face; diffuse expiratory wheezes; skin showing 4-cm diameter raised white lesions with surrounding erythema that are intensely pruritic; edema involving the entire right arm.

Labs CBC/Lytes: normal. Tryptase level: 40 ng/mL (normal <10)

Imaging None.

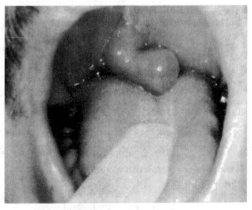

Figure 5-1. Marked angioedema of the uvula and soft palate.

9

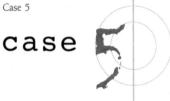

case 5

Hymenoptera Hypersensitivity

Pathogenesis

Hymenoptera hypersensitivity is a life-threatening reaction that results from a **systemic reaction to the sting from a flying insect.** Patients with specific IgE against a member of the **hymenoptera family (honey bee, yellow jacket, paper wasp, yellow-faced and white-faced hornet)** are at risk of developing a systemic allergic reaction when stung by these insects. Exposure to the antigenic protein (found in hymenoptera venom) elicits mast cell degranulation with the release of preformed mediators (histamine, **tryptase)** as well as synthesis of leukotrienes and prostaglandins. Histamine leads to the development of hives and edema. **Histamine, leukotrienes, and prostaglandins** also cause throat constriction due to laryngeal edema as well as bronchospasm. Gastric histamine receptors cause abdominal discomfort and nausea. The widespread histamine release leads to third-spacing of fluids and resultant hypotension (hypovolemic shock). History of recent sting by a flying insect strongly suggests the diagnosis.

Epidemiology

Approximately 3% of the US population is estimated to have had a reaction to venom of insects in the order Hymenoptera. The annual death rate from these reactions is 40 adults per year. Onset is rapid with early symptoms occurring within minutes, and most patients present within 1 hour of the sting.

Management

Prompt administration of **epinephrine** intramuscularly. Additional treatment includes IV fluids, **H1- (diphenhydramine) and H2- (ranitidine) antihistamines, systemic corticosteroids, and nebulized β2 receptor agonists (albuterol).** Pressors can be used for refractory hypotension. Patients should be prescribed an **epinephrine autoinjector** (Epipen) and should undergo **hymenoptera skin testing.** All patients who have had a systemic reaction to hymenoptera should receive **immunotherapy.**

Complications

Death from anaphylactic shock occurs in 40 adults in the U.S. each year.

Breakout Point

- Elevated tryptase level
- Prescribe an Epipen

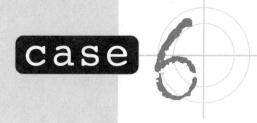

case 6

ID/CC   A **35-year-old caucasian** man presents with **profound flushing** of his face with drinking **alcoholic** beverages.

HPI   The patient has noticed this flushing sensation for several years with ingestion of any alcohol, often after only one drink. This flushing has also occurred with exercise. He further notes **severe abdominal discomfort** at times. He has had **anaphylactic reactions to bee stings** in the past and had one episode without a clear cause. He has also experienced a number of **syncopal episodes** over the years. He is allergic to morphine and vancomycin, both of which cause hives and flushing. Over the years he has found a number of **small, yellow-tan to reddish-brown lesions** on his skin that develop hives around them if scratched.

PE   VS: normal. PE: well-appearing, abdominal exam reveals hepatosplenomegaly; general lymphadenopathy; skin with small, reddish-brown slightly raised papules mostly found on the trunk with sparing of the palms, soles and face; scratching at the lesions causes hives with surrounding erythema at the site of the lesion **(Darier sign).**

Labs   CBC/Lytes normal. Urine: 24-hour urine collection for 5-hydroxyindoleacetic acid (5-HIAA) and metanephrines is negative. Tryptase level: 30 ng/mL (normal <10). Bone marrow aspiration: >15 mast cells in aggregate that are tryptase positive. A c-kit mutation was found.

Imaging   Technitium-99 scan: multiple erosive lesions predominantly in the long bones.

11

case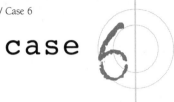

Mastocytosis

Pathogenesis

Systemic mastocytosis is caused by an **activating mutation in c-kit** that enables the **proliferation of mast cells and prolongs their survival**. The increased burden of mast cells leads to elevated levels of histamine, tryptase, tumor necrosis factor-α, prostaglandin D2, leukotrienes, and platelet activating factor. The **urticaria pigmentosa lesions** have high levels of mast cells. The increased histamine production leads to the local urticaria on stroking these lesions. It also causes **dyspepsia** through increased gastric acid secretion via gastric histamine receptors.

Epidemiology

Prevalence unknown but reported to be 1/1,000–8,000 new visits to a dermatology clinic. It occurs at any age. There is no gender predominance.

Management

Oral cromolyn sodium solution is used for control of abdominal symptoms. **H1- and H2-receptor antagonists** are used on an as-needed basis for hives and dyspepsia. **Epinephrine autoinjectors** can be used in case of hypotensive episodes.

Complications

Often follows an indolent cource with episodic reactions. Some cases evolve to mastocytosis with an associated hematologic disorder which dictates long term survival.

Breakout Point

- Darier's sign on exam
- Urticaria pigmentosa
- Elevated tryptase level
- Can evolve to leukemia

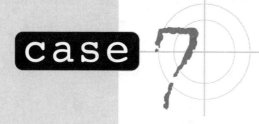

ID/CC An **11-month old white boy** is brought to the ER by his mother with **facial erythema, lip swelling,** and **wheezing.**

HPI His mother reports that he had just eaten his brother's **peanut butter** cracker. Although she had not given him any peanut-containing foods before, she did eat peanuts during her pregnancy and while she was breast-feeding. Within a few minutes, she noticed redness of her son's face that progressed to lip swelling. She gave him some liquid diphenhydramine (Benadryl), but his symptoms did not improve, and he began to wheeze.

PE VS: afebrile, tachycardia (HR 140), tachypnea (RR 24), O_2 saturation 86% on room air. PE: crying, flushing of the face with lip swelling and perioral cyanosis; diffuse expiratory wheezes; skin with areas of eczema.

Labs CBC/Lytes: normal. Radioallergosorbent test (RAST) for peanut (detects antigen-specific IgE antibodies): positive.

Imaging None.

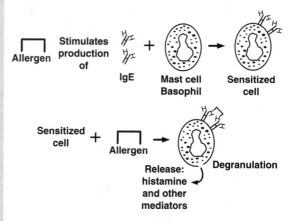

Figure 7-1. Mechanisms of IgE-mediated food allergy.

13

case 7

Peanut Allergy

Pathogenesis

Sensitization to peanut allergen (IgE-mediated or non-IgE mediated) often **occurs very early in life, including in utero or during breast-feeding.** In children, **egg, peanut, milk, soy, wheat, and fish** account for 85% to 90% of food-related allergic reactions.

Epidemiology

Approximately 1% of infants develop a peanut allergy, and only about 20% of these children outgrow their peanut allergy. Most infants have their first allergic reaction to peanuts by an average age of 22 months. Milk is the most common food allergy among children, followed by egg allergy, then peanut allergy.

Management

If a child is found to be allergic to peanuts (usually by RAST or skin testing), **strict avoidance is critical. Yearly RAST testing** can be performed to see if the child is likely to **outgrow peanut allergy.**

Complications

Anaphylaxis is a common complication if strict avoidance is not adhered to risk factors for fatal anaphylaxis include: not receiving epinephrine soon enough, history of asthma, and having prior episodes of anaphylaxis.

Breakout Point

- Strict avoidance of peanuts
- RAST skin testing
- Must carry an Epipen

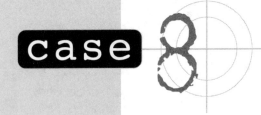

case 8

ID/CC   A **32-year-old pregnant woman** with a history of penicillin allergy is diagnosed with syphilis.

HPI   She describes a maculopapular rash to penicillin for an ear infection at the age of 21 years. She has avoided all beta-lactams since this reaction occurred and has been told never to take penicillin again. She is now 28 weeks pregnant and has been diagnosed with primary syphilis.

PE   VS: tachycardia (HR 110). PE: genitals with primary syphilitic lesion.

Labs   CBC/Lytes: normal. RPR/VDRL positive. Skin test was positive to penicillin when she was 21 years of age.

Imaging   US of fetus: normal for gestation.

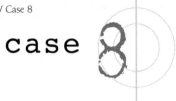

case 8

Penicillin Allergy

Pathogenesis

Penicillin allergy is the **most common cause of allergic drug reactions and anaphylaxis.** Penicillin is simple in structure and of low molecular weight. These low-molecular-weight structures, or **haptens,** cause an immune response by binding to native proteins in the plasma and cell surfaces to form hapten-carrier complexes. These complexes form antigens that IgE on mast cells can recognize. The IgE is cross-linked by the hapten complexes, leading to mast cell release of histamine causing **pruritus, hives, angioedema, and/or anaphylaxis.**

Epidemiology

Ten percent of the population claims to be allergic to penicillin, but in reality, only 1% to 3% have an IgE-mediated response to penicillin. Anaphylactic reactions occur most often in adults 20–49 years of age.

Management

Aztreonam is a safe alternative in patients who are allergic to beta-lactams. In clinical situations requiring penicillin treatment, a penicillin-allergic patient may successfully receive penicillin by a desensitization protocol. Historically, skin testing was performed to the major and minor determinants of penicillin G and the specific beta-lactam to be given to the patient. If skin testing was positive, beta-lactams were avoided. The major determinant is no longer available in the United States, so skin testing is no longer available. The current standards of care are a **graded challenge** (low-risk patients, remote history of a rash in childhood), **avoidance,** or **desensitization** (high-risk patients, skin test–positive patients) in those with beta-lactam allergy who absolutely need to be treated with a beta-lactam. Cephalosporins share the beta-lactam ring with penicillins. First-generation cephalosporins have about 10% cross-reactivity, and third-generation cephalosporins carry a 2% to 5% cross-reactivity; thus, **cephalosporins should be avoided** in these patients. **Meropenem should also be avoided** because of an estimated 50% cross-reactivity.

Complications

There are approximately 400 fatalities annually from penicillin allergy and anaphylaxis.

Breakout Point

- Aztreonam is tolerated in patients allergic to beta-lactams
- There is 5% to 10% cross-reactivity between penicillin and cephalosporins
- Desensitization can be used to give beta-lactams to patients who are skin test–positive

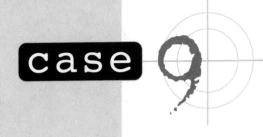

case

ID/CC   A **5-month-old Asian boy** presents to the GI clinic with diarrhea and failure to thrive.

HPI   The boy was the product of a full-term pregnancy by **consanguineous parents.** He **initially grew well** but, beginning at the age of 3 months, started to move from the 25th percentile for weight to the 3rd percentile. He has had **two episodes of otitis media** treated with antibiotics and developed **diarrhea** on both occasions that was labeled as antibiotic-associated diarrhea. He developed **pneumonia** at the age of 5 months and was treated by his pediatrician with another course of antibiotics. He again developed diarrhea in the past week, and his parents thought that he had begun coughing more lately.

PE   VS: febrile, tachycardic, normotensive. PE: thin, small for stated age; sunken anterior fontanelle; absent tonsils, no palpable lymph nodes; rhonchi at the left base; abdomen soft without hepatosplenomegaly.

Labs   CBC: WBC 3,000. IgG 150 mg/dL (low), IgA 10 mg/dL (low), IgM 10 mg/dL (low). T cells (CD3) undetectable. B cells (CD19) normal. Natural killer (NK) cells (CD56) undetectable.

Imaging   CXR: left lower lobe pneumonia. Absent thymic shadow.

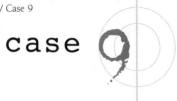

case 9

Severe Combined Immunodeficiency

Pathogenesis

X-linked severe combined immunodeficiency (X-SCID) is a profound primary immunodeficiency. Patients have an **abnormal gene for the common gamma chain,** which is found on **IL receptors for IL-2, IL-4, IL-7, IL-9, IL-15, and IL-21.** The inability to signal through these receptors leads to **failure to develop T cells or NK cells.** Most patients with X-SCID **have B cells, but these cells are unable to form antibodies and cannot respond to vaccinations.** Without an immune system, these children are at risk for developing bacterial, viral, and opportunistic infections, leading to overwhelming sepsis and death.

Epidemiology

SCID is estimated to occur in 1 of 50,000 to 100,000 live births. **X-SCID is the most common form of SCID** and accounts for 46% of all cases.

Management

X-SCID is a medical emergency. Bone marrow transplantation before the age of $3^1/2$ months offers a 97% chance of survival. Most patients require IVIG for life.

Complications

Death from infections usually occurs before two years of age in patients who do not receive a bone marrow transplant. There is an increased risk of developing cancers later in life.

Breakout Point

- X-SCID due to abnormal common gamma chain gene
- T and B cell defect
- Presents as failure to thrive
- Bone marrow transplant early

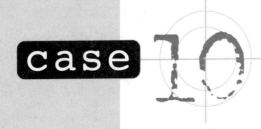

case 10

ID/CC   A **68-year-old white man** who works as a **farmer** complains of several discrete dry, rough, scaly lesions on his **forehead**.

HPI   He has worked **outdoors** for many years and has **never used sunscreen**. He states that he first noticed the lesions several months ago but adds that they are not painful unless he runs his fingers over them.

PE   VS: normal. PE: **fair-skinned** with **blond hair** and **blue eyes**; numerous, small (<1 cm), coarse, yellow-brown lesions with reddish tinge on forehead, ears, posterior neck, and dorsal aspect of hands (sun-exposed regions).

Labs   None.

Imaging   None.

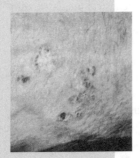

Figure 10-1. Superficial flattened papules covered by a dry scale; often multiple; round or irregular; pink, tan, or gray colored.

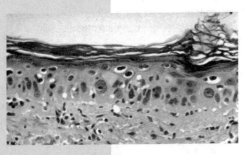

Figure 10-2. High-power microscopy shows **atypical basal epidermal pleomorphic keratinocytes**.

case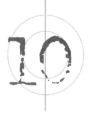

Actinic Keratosis

Pathogenesis

Actinic or solar keratosis results from repeated and prolonged exposure to UV light (primarily UVB, 290 to 320 nm), ionizing radiation, or polycyclic aromatic hydrocarbons and arsenicals, leading to damage to keratinocytes. Clonal expansion of mutated forms of the tumor suppressor gene p53 has been observed in cases of both actinic keratosis and SCC, indicating that actinic keratosis is a premalignant lesion that may be regarded as SCC in situ.

Epidemiology

Actinic keratosis, like SCC of the skin, occurs with increased frequency among **males,** individuals with a **light complexion,** those who **work outdoors,** people who frequent tanning salons, and individuals from Australia or the southwestern United States; the disease is rarely seen in blacks or East Indians. Immunosuppressed patients are also at increased risk.

Management

The initial treatment of uncomplicated lesions involves the **topical application of 5-FU and/or liquid nitrogen.** A **skin biopsy** may be necessary to rule out SCC if evidence of ulceration or induration is present. Extensive skin involvement or evidence of nodular lesions requires **surgical excision.** Prevention primarily involves the use of **UVA/UVB sunscreens.**

Complications

Approximately 1 in 1,000 solar keratosis lesions develop into invasive SCC each year.

Breakout Point

- Pink, sandpapery, tender patches
- Precancerous lesion, can develop into SCC of the skin
- Prevalent in elderly, fair-skinned patients on sun-exposed areas
- Treated with 5-FU cream or surgery

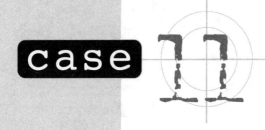

case 11

ID/CC	A **44-year-old man** complains of **sore, scaly hands.**
HPI	The patient states that he has worked as a **bricklayer** (chronic exposure to chromate salts in cement) for the past 20 years. He adds that the condition of his hands has gradually worsened over the past year.
PE	VS: normal. PE: bilateral hyperkeratosis, maceration, fissuring, and erosion of palms and proximal portion of each digit.
Labs	**Patch test** elicits a local response at a distant site.
Imaging	None.

case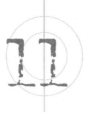

Contact Dermatitis

Pathogenesis | Contact dermatitis appears in two forms: **nonallergic** (caused by chemical irritation) and **allergic/eczematous (type IV hypersensitivity reaction to an antigen)**. Acids and bases cause irritant contact dermatitis, whereas poison ivy and oak usually cause allergic contact dermatitis. Irritant contact dermatitis is concentration dependent and does not require sensitization (unlike allergic contact dermatitis, which depends on sensitization). Lesions are sharply marginated. Chronic toxic or irritant dermatitis results from repeated exposure to agents that gradually erode the barrier function of the skin and ultimately elicit an inflammatory response.

Epidemiology | Occupational exposures play a crucial role in the etiology of contact dermatitis. Young children only infrequently present with allergic contact dermatitis, and black individuals appear to be less susceptible.

Management | **Removal of offending agent; topical steroids.** Additionally, one may drain large vesicles without uncovering them and apply wet dressings with Burow's solution every 3 hours for acute dermatitis.

Breakout Point |
- Occurs within 24–96 hours of exposure
- Type IV delayed type hypersensitivity
- Causes: poison ivy, poison oak, poison sumac, nickel, potassium dichromate (cements), ethylenediamine (dyes)

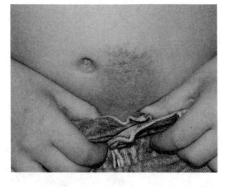

Figure 11-1. Reaction in area of contact with rubber or nickel in clothes; note skin sparing where contact was not made (a different case).

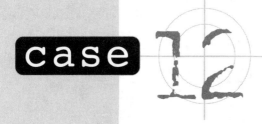

ID/CC A **32-year-old man** presents with an intensely **pruritic vesiculopapular** eruption limited to the extensor surfaces of his knees and elbows.

HPI The patient reports **repeated episodes** of the rash over the past few years. The first episode occurred at 24 years of age.

PE VS: normal. PE: cardiopulmonary exam normal; pruritic vesiculopapular eruption on extensor surfaces of knees and elbows; remainder of exam normal.

Labs Direct immunofluorescence of normal perilesional skin demonstrates granular deposits of IgA in papillary dermis and along epidermal basement membrane zone; no circulating IgA.

Imaging None.

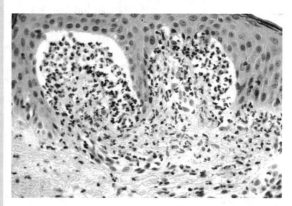

Figure 12-1. Cutaneous lesion of dermal papillary abscesses of neutrophils with vesicle formation at the dermal–epidermal junction.

DERMATOLOGY

23

case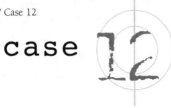

Dermatitis Herpetiformis

Pathogenesis

Dermatitis herpetiformis is an idiopathic autoimmune disease characterized by **granular deposits of IgA** in the papillary dermis and along the epidermal basement membrane zone with intensely pruritic, chronic vesiculopapular lesions symmetrically distributed over the extensor surfaces.

Epidemiology

More than 90% of patients with dermatitis herpetiformis are **HLA-B8/DRw3 and HLA-DQw2 positive.** Almost all have associated, usually subclinical, **gluten-sensitive enteropathy.**

Management

Maintenance of a **gluten-free diet** may diminish outbreaks. **Dapsone** should be used in exacerbations.

Breakout Point

- Associated with gluten enteropathy/celiac sprue
- Granular IgA deposits in dermal papillae
- Treated by avoiding gluten

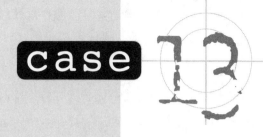

ID/CC	A **23-year-old woman** presents to the clinic complaining of painful, tender nodules on the anterior surface of her legs.
HPI	She had a **fever** and **sore throat** prior to the appearance of the lesions. She also complains of an **aching pain in her ankles.**
PE	VS: **fever** (38.6°C). PE: **numerous** erythematous, round lesions 3–20 cm in diameter that are poorly demarcated and located on lower legs bilaterally; palpable nodules that are indurated and tender.
Labs	ESR elevated; throat culture positive for GABHS.
Imaging	CXR: normal.

DERMATOLOGY

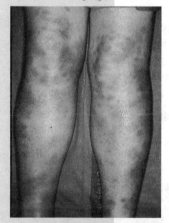

Figure 13-1. Erythematous nodules on the anterior shins bilaterally.

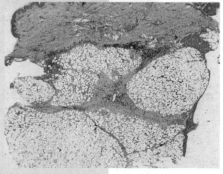

Figure 13-2. Inflammation in the upper subcutis with thickened septa.

case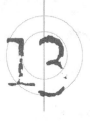

Erythema Nodosum

Pathogenesis

Erythema nodosum is an acute inflammatory or immunologic disorder leading to a septal panniculitis in subcutaneous fat. It arises in **response to infectious agents** (eg, GABHS, *Yersinia*, histoplasmosis, **coccidioidomycosis**, and TB), in **inflammatory conditions** such as sarcoidosis and **ulcerative colitis**, and in response to **drugs** such as sulfonamides and OCPs. Generally, the condition remits spontaneously within 6 weeks.

Epidemiology

The most common cause of acute panniculitis. Patients are generally **female** (3:1) and **between 15 and 30 years of age.**

Management

Treat the underlying cause and initiate supportive measures such as bed rest, decreased weight bearing, compressive bandages, and/or NSAIDs. In severe cases where infectious agents have been ruled out, prednisone may be administered.

Complications

Complications are related to the underlying disease.

Breakout Point

- Painful red nodules on shins of young women
- Associated with infection, inflammation, and drugs
- Most common skin manifestation of sarcoidosis

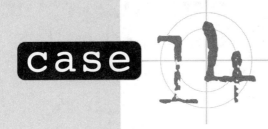

ID/CC A **34-year-old homosexual man** presents with unusual **purple-red, painless skin lesions** on the face and neck.

HPI He also complains of shortness of breath and adds that he has had dull chest pain and a limited appetite and has **coughed up blood** on a few occasions (HEMOPTYSIS). He has been **HIV-positive** for 6 years.

PE VS: normal. PE: pallor; mucocutaneous **purplish macules;** palpable abdominal masses and tenderness; generalized indurated lymphadenopathy; pedal edema.

Labs CBC: anemia; thrombocytosis; lymphopenia. **CD4 lymphocyte count decreased** biopsy of lesion reveals **proliferation of spindle cells, endothelial cells,** and extravasation of RBCs.

Imaging CXR: bilateral lower lobe infiltrates obscure the margins of the mediastinum and diaphragm (finding suggestive of **pulmonary metastases).** Fiberoptic bronchoscopy and endoscopy for visualization and biopsy of other suspected sites should be performed. CT chest and bone scan stages the tumor.

DERMATOLOGY

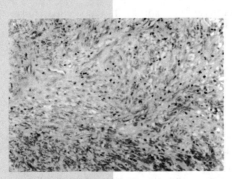

Figure 14-1. Spindle cell proliferation with slit-like vascular spaces.

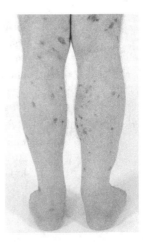

Figure 14-2. Multiple mucocutaneous **purplish macules.**

case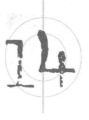

Kaposi's Sarcoma

Pathogenesis

KS is a **hemangiosarcoma** that may affect the skin, viscera, and mucous membranes. The lymph nodes, GI tract, and lungs are also commonly involved. KS is usually seen as an "opportunistic" neoplasm in HIV-positive homosexual men but may be seen during any stage of the infection. Etiologic associations include KS-associated virus (HHV-8).

Epidemiology

KS in a male younger than 60 years is strongly suggestive of HIV infection. Ninety-six percent of AIDS-related cases occur in homosexual men. KS is rare in children and in hemophiliacs with AIDS.

Management

Optimize control of HIV infection with effective anti-retroviral therapy. Local therapy includes radiation therapy, intralesional vinblastine, cryotherapy and topical retinoids for cutaneous lesions, and **resection of isolated lung metastases.** Few AIDS patients with KS die as a result of this malignancy; thus, treatment regimens that suppress the immune system should be avoided. Treatment may be indicated for lesions that are associated with significant discomfort (eg, those located over a joint), dysphagia (eg, oropharyngeal lesions), or cosmetic problems (eg, facial lesions). **Interferon** is useful in early disease. **Combination chemotherapy** with doxorubicin, etoposide, vinblastine, and bleomycin is warranted in aggressive KS. Prognosis is related to CD4 count and immune status.

Complications

Ulceration of the cutaneous lesion with subsequent infection is a common side effect of therapy; GI obstruction and hemorrhage may occur with internal lesions.

Breakout Point

- Is an AIDS-defining illness
- Is likely caused by coinfection of HHV-8
- Common site of lesions is lower extremities, head, neck, and mucous membranes, but they can occur anywhere

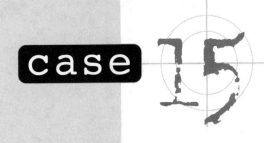

case 15

ID/CC	An **18-year-old man** presents with **scaly salmon-pink lesions** on the extensor surfaces of his elbows and knees.
HPI	The patient is otherwise healthy.
PE	VS: normal. PE: **erythematous papules and plaques** with silver scaling on extensor surfaces of elbows and knees; nail pitting of hands.
Labs	Skin biopsy shows focal parakeratosis, hyperkeratosis, elongation and thickening of rete ridges, and thinning of epidermis above dermal papillae.
Imaging	None.

DERMATOLOGY

case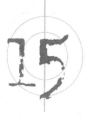

Psoriasis

Pathogenesis

Psoriasis is an idiopathic disease, perhaps autoimmune in origin, that is characterized by epidermal proliferation with **increased thickness of the stratum spinosum** (ACANTHOSIS), **retention of nuclei in the cells of the stratum corneum** (PARAKERATOSIS), and collections of neutrophils (MONRO MICROABSCESSES) within the stratum corneum; it most often involves the **extensor surfaces** of the elbows and knees, scalp, and sacral areas.

Epidemiology

Psoriasis is a common dermatologic disease. Thirty-five percent of patients have a family history of psoriasis.

Management

Mild to moderate psoriasis can be treated with **topical corticosteroids. Keratolytic agents** (eg, salicylic acid) can be used when marked hyperkeratosis is present. **Topical retinoids** or **tar compounds** may be beneficial when alternated with corticosteroids. Severe psoriasis should be treated **chemotherapeutically** (methotrexate, cyclosporin) and with **UV light.**

Complications

Extensive disease can lead to **psoriatic arthritis.** Secondary bacterial infection may occur as well (pustular psoriasis).

Breakout Point

- Autoimmune disease associated with increased T-cell activity
- Plaques covered by silvery white scale
- Associated with pits in nails and yellowing of nails
- Development of psoriatic arthritis in hands and feet in 10% of patients

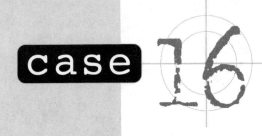

case 16

ID/CC	A **74-year-old man** with Parkinson disease presents with a greasy, **scaly rash** that has spread from his scalp to his eyebrows, eyelids, and nasolabial folds.
HPI	The patient reports increased itching over the involved areas. He has been treated for severe dandruff in the past year.
PE	VS: normal. PE: bilateral, symmetrically distributed patches of greasy, erythematous scales localized to hair-covered areas of the head and nasolabial folds.
Labs	None.
Imaging	None.

case  16

Seborrheic Dermatitis

Pathogenesis

Seborrheic dermatitis is a common, chronic disorder characterized by **greasy scales** overlying erythematous plaques or patches. Lesions are most commonly located on the scalp (may be recognized as severe dandruff) but may also affect the eyebrows, eyelids, glabella, nasolabial folds, or ears. Although the condition is more frequently seen in patients with Parkinson disease, CVA, or HIV, the majority of individuals with seborrheic dermatitis have no underlying disorder. Its etiology is thought to be an inflammatory reaction to the yeast *Pityrosporum.*

Epidemiology

Seborrheic dermatitis may be evident in the first weeks of life, commonly affecting the scalp (CRADLE CAP). It is rarely seen in children after infancy but is evident again in adulthood. It affects approximately 3% of the general population.

Management

Treat the scalp with 2.5% selenium sulfide, zinc pyrithione, tar, salicylic acid, or ketoconazole shampoo. Apply **low-dose corticosteroids** or **ketoconazole** cream to the affected skin in severe cases.

Breakout Point

- Associated with the yeast *Pityrosporum (Malassezia furfur)*
- Greasy scaling over red inflamed skin found on scalp, face, postauricular areas, and trunk
- Waxing and waning severity
- May worsen in Parkinson disease or AIDS

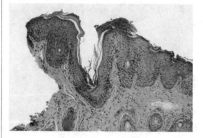

Figure 16-1. Characteristic neutrophilic keratosis, hyperplastic epidermis.

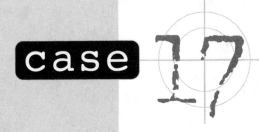

ID/CC A **63-year-old white man** presents with a **reddish nodule** on the left side of his lip that has failed to heal for several months.

HPI The patient reports a **tendency to sunburn** due to his fair skin. He had another lesion in the same location that was diagnosed as **actinic keratosis** almost 10 years ago. The present lesion is not painful or pruritic.

PE VS: normal. PE: blond and **fair-skinned**; no acute distress; HEENT remarkable for 1 × 1 cm **red, conical, hard nodule with ulceration** on superior aspect of lower left lip margin.

Labs None.

Imaging **Biopsy** of lesion reveals invasion of dermis by sheets and islands of neoplastic epidermal cells.

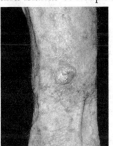

Figure 17-1. Reddish-white nodule on the skin.

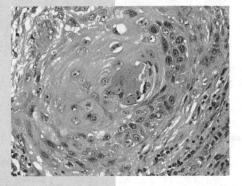

Figure 17-2. Biopsy of lesion reveals invasion of dermis by sheets and islands of neoplastic epidermal cells, often with **"keratin pearls."**

DERMATOLOGY

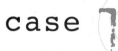 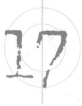

Squamous Cell Carcinoma

Pathogenesis

SCC is a malignant neoplasm of keratinizing epithelial cells. It may develop anywhere on the body but typically involves sun-damaged skin. Several premalignant forms should be noted, including actinic keratosis, actinic cheilitis, and Bowen disease (may develop into SCC in 20% of cases).

Epidemiology

Nonmelanoma skin cancer is the most common cancer in the United States, with more than 800,000 cases diagnosed each year; SCC accounts for approximately 20% of cases (basal cell carcinoma accounts for 70% to 80%). The causes are multifactorial, including **cumulative exposure to UVB sunlight**, male sex, older age, Celtic ancestry, fair complexion, tendency to sunburn, and outdoor occupation. As many as 45% of patients with renal transplants develop SCC within 10 years.

Management

Surgical excision is the mainstay of treatment; Mohs microsurgery, radiation, and cryosurgery are alternate modalities. Metastases are treated with lymph node dissection, irradiation, or both. Because most cases are related to chronic UVB exposure, emphasis should be placed on prevention with regular use of **sunscreens** and protective clothing. Close follow-up for detection of recurrence, metastasis, or new cancers is indicated in all patients with a history of skin cancer.

Complications

SCC carries a **low but significant malignant potential.** Metastases occur in 5% to 10% of patients with cutaneous lesions, 11% of ear lesions, and 13% of lower lip lesions; the rate of metastasis is higher for cancers arising in burn scars, chronic ulcerations, genitalia, and recurrent tumors. Regional lymph nodes are the most common site of metastasis. The prognosis is poor in patients with metastatic disease.

Breakout Point

- Presents as nonhealing ulcer or nodule (telangiectasic pearly papule is basal cell carcinoma)
- Can metastasize (unlike basal cell carcinoma)
- Second most common skin cancer (after basal cell carcinoma)
- Histologically characterized by keratin pearls

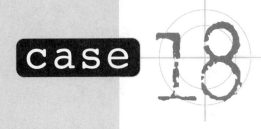

case 18

ID/CC	A **40-year-old man** complains of high, intermittent, spiking **fever with chills, RUQ abdominal pain,** malaise, anorexia, and nausea of 1 week's duration.
HPI	He is a missionary who just returned from a 3-year stay in **rural South America**. Directed questioning reveals that he suffered from **diarrhea with blood and mucus** (DYSENTERY) as well as tenesmus on several occasions (due to intestinal amebiasis). He additionally reports a 4-kg weight loss over the past 2 months.
PE	VS: **fever** (39.3°C); tachycardia (HR 110); normal BP. PE: pallor; slight jaundice; no lymphadenopathy; right lung field shows **diminished breath sounds and basilar rales;** soft tissue edema and shiny appearance over RUQ with **marked, tender hepatomegaly;** no ascites, spider angiomata, or caput medusae.
Labs	CBC: **anemia** (Hb 10.4); marked **leukocytosis** (18,350); **neutrophilia** (89%). Elevated ESR; **amebic trophozoites and ova in stool** (positivity rate of 10%–30%); chocolate-colored ("anchovy sauce") pus obtained by needle aspiration of abscess does not show parasites (positivity rate is <30%; amebae are confined to the periphery of lesion); positive complement fixation test reaction to *Entamoeba histolytica*.
Imaging	XR, abdomen: an air-fluid level is seen in the right subphrenic abscess.

INFECTIOUS DISEASE

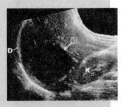

Figure 18-1. US, abdomen: a large hypoechoic mass (1) is seen in the liver in another patient; note the diaphragm (D) and kidney (K).

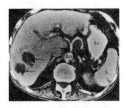

Figure 18-2. CT, abdomen: a different case in which two areas of low attenuation are seen in the right lobe of the liver.

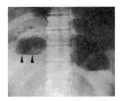

Figure 18-3. XR, abdomen: an air-fluid level is seen in this right subphrenic abscess (the normal gastric bubble is seen on the left).

case 18

Amebic Liver Abscess

Pathogenesis

Amebic abscess of the liver is a complication of intestinal infection with *Entamoeba histolytica*. A history of prior travel to an endemic area plus the triad of **fever, hepatomegaly,** and **RUQ pain** are characteristics of hepatic amebic abscess.

Epidemiology

The liver is the most common extraintestinal location of amebiasis; prior intestinal infection may be asymptomatic or may present as amebic dysentery. The abscess is usually **single** and more commonly presents in the posterosuperior surface of the **right lobe of the liver.** It shows a **male predominance.**

Management

Metronidazole is the mainstay of therapy and is usually given with iodoquinol as a luminal amebicide. Dehydroemetine may be used for resistant cases and may be followed by chloroquine. Most abscesses respond to medical therapy. Attempt **percutaneous aspiration/surgical drainage** for imminent rupture, large abscesses, location in the left lobe (danger of pericardial rupture), secondary bacterial infection, or failure of medical treatment. Rule out hydatidiform disease (ECHINOCOCCOSIS) before attempting aspiration.

Complications

Secondary pyogenic infection is the most common complication. **Rupture** may be life-threatening. Involvement of the psoas and gluteus muscle, pararectal spaces, spleen, or brain may occur by contiguity or metastatic dissemination.

Breakout Point

- Triad of fever, hepatomegaly, and RUQ pain
- Caused by *Entamoeba histolytica* (protozoal parasite)
- Do not aspirate abscess until rule out *Echinococcus* (aspirating echinococcal cyst is associated with anaphylactic shock)
- Prevalent in travelers to Central and South America, Asia, and Africa

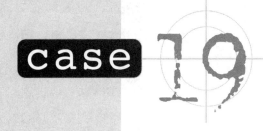

case 19

ID/CC	A **45-year-old man** with bronchial **asthma** complains of a **productive cough.**
HPI	He also complains of progressively increasing breathlessness with intermittent attacks of severe dyspnea. He notes the presence of **brownish plugs** in his sputum.
PE	VS: **tachypnea** (RR 28). PE: mild respiratory distress; mild **cyanosis**; pallor; occasional rhonchi and wheezes heard bilaterally; **clubbing** of fingernails.
Labs	CBC: **eosinophilia.** Skin testing reveals immediate reaction to *Aspergillus fumigatus*; serum IgG to *A. fumigatus* present; serum IgE elevated; sputum culture grows *A. fumigatus.*
Imaging	CXR: branching, fingerlike shadows from mucoid impaction of dilated bronchi.

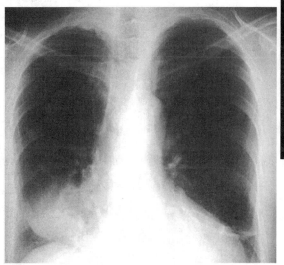

Figure 19-1. CXR: branching, fingerlike shadows from mucoid impaction of dilated bronchi.

case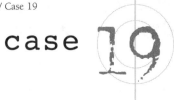

Aspergillosis: Allergic

Pathogenesis	**Allergic bronchopulmonary aspergillosis (ABPA)** is characterized by preexisting asthma accompanied by eosinophilia, IgE antibody to *Aspergillus*, and fleeting finger-shaped pulmonary infiltrates on CXR.
Epidemiology	ABPA is usually seen in atopic asthmatic individuals 20 to 40 years of age.
Management	Allergen avoidance along with symptomatic management with **corticosteroids** and treatment of underlying lung disease (bronchodilators) are indicated. Systemic **antifungal therapy is not effective** in endobronchial disease.
Complications	*Aspergillus* may occasionally colonize a preexisting pulmonary cavity and produce an aspergilloma, which may be complicated by hemoptysis and should be treated by lobectomy. **Invasive aspergillosis** may occur in immunocompromised patients.
Breakout Point	<ul><li>ABPA is a hypersensitivity reaction to *A. fumigatus* colonization in bronchi</li><li>Aspergilloma is a fungus ball (mycetoma) that develops in a preexisting cavity in lung parenchyma</li><li>ABPA is diagnosed in patients with asthma, eosinophilia, elevated IgE level, and positive skin and antibody tests to *Aspergillus* fumigates</li></ul>

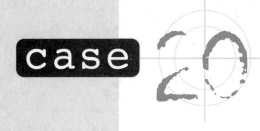

ID/CC A **28-year-old man** is brought to the ER complaining
of sudden-onset **double vision**, hoarseness, **slurred
speech**, and **difficulty swallowing** for the past few
hours.

HPI He also reports repeated vomiting and **symmetric
weakness** of the extremities that has **progressed cau-
dally**. Directed questioning reveals that he ate some
home-canned stew yesterday.

PE VS: **no fever**; postural hypotension. PE: **alert** but in
acute distress; severe abdominal tenderness; bowel
sounds depressed; ocular exam reveals **ptosis, dilated
pupils sluggishly reacting to light**, and extraocular
muscle paresis (type A may have no ocular signs);
DTRs depressed in proportion to weakness.

Labs Blood positive for *Clostridium botulinum* toxin. PFTs:
spirometry reveals normal vital capacity (to rule out
respiratory muscle weakness).

Imaging None.

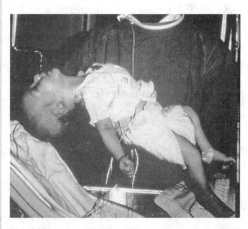

Figure 20-1. Floppy baby syndrome characterized by marked
loss of muscle tone (a different case of the same diagnosis).

INFECTIOUS DISEASE

case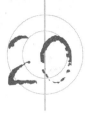

Botulism

Pathogenesis	Botulism is an acute **descending paralytic disease** that **begins in the cranial nerves** and **descends caudally** to affect the extremities (without sensory deficits). Botulinum toxin **blocks acetylcholine release** in motor nerve terminals, resulting in a **flaccid paralysis.** Autonomic nerve endings may also be affected, resulting in dry mouth, constipation, or urine retention. Cases may be classified as **food-borne** botulism (derived from contaminated food), **wound** botulism (from localized toxin production), **infant** botulism (ingestion and/or gut production in infants), **adult–infant** botulism (similar to infants, but affecting older children and adults), or indeterminate. **Botulism should be considered only in afebrile-oriented patients who have a descending paralysis.**
Epidemiology	Botulism occurs worldwide. Of the eight known types of *C. botulinum* toxins (types A–G), types A, B, and E commonly cause disease in humans. Food-borne illness is associated with **home-canned vegetables, fruit, and condiments** (infant poisoning is associated with contaminated honey). This type of botulism occurs when contaminated food is preserved with **spores** or when food is not heated to a temperature that destroys the **toxin.**
Management	**Equine antitoxin** emergently while monitoring the patient for anaphylaxis and serum sickness. Emetic and gastric lavage may be useful if ingestion of contaminated food is recent. Infant botulism is not helped by antibiotics. Antibiotics that act at the neuromuscular junctions **(aminoglycosides) should be avoided.** Monitor spirometry, pulse oximetry, and ABGs to guard against **respiratory failure.** If vital capacity falls to less than 30%, intubation and **mechanical ventilation** are required, especially if paralysis, hypercarbia, and hypoxemia are progressing.
Complications	Fatalities from botulism poisoning are low due to the availability of respiratory support. Artificial respiration may be required for weeks in severe cases, and residual autonomic dysfunction may be observed.
Breakout Point	• *Clostridium botulinum* is a gram-positive rod • Toxin blocks presynaptic acetylcholine release • Ingestion of home-canned goods or honey, IV drug use • Symmetric, descending motor paralysis in an alert patient with intact sensation

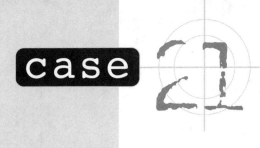

ID/CC   A **35-year-old man** with **AIDS** complains of **diminution of vision** in his right eye.

HPI   The patient states that he sees **floaters** and acknowledges a recent **fever.**

PE   VS: **fever** (38.6°C). PE: funduscopic exam demonstrates **perivascular hemorrhagic exudates** and necrotic areas in right eye; decreased visual acuity.

Labs   CD4 count <50.

Imaging   None.

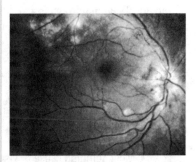

Figure 21-1. Fundascopic perivascular white infiltrates with retinal hemorrhage.

INFECTIOUS DISEASE

case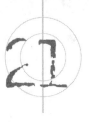

Cytomegalovirus Retinitis

Pathogenesis
CMV retinitis arises following **reactivation of a latent infection,** most commonly in AIDS patients with CD4 counts <100. It causes progressive **necrotizing retinitis** that eventually leads to blindness.

Epidemiology
CMV is common; more than 50% of adults have antibodies to the virus, and more than 90% of homosexual men have **latent infections.** CMV retinitis is the most common opportunistic eye infection in HIV patients.

Management
Treatment may be local (to the affected eye alone), systemic, or a combination of both. Treatment options include IV **ganciclovir,** foscarnet, and cidofovir; oral ganciclovir; intravitreous injection of ganciclovir, foscarnet, and fomivirsen; and surgically implanted slow-release ganciclovir devices.

Complications
Retinal detachment and blindness, line sepsis from IV drug administration, and CMV involvement of the contralateral eye or other end-organ involvement (pneumonitis, colitis, encephalitis).

Breakout Point

- Most common cause of visual loss in patients with AIDS
- White infiltrates with retinal hemorrhage ("cheese pizza" appearance) along retinal vessels
- Treat with ganciclovir

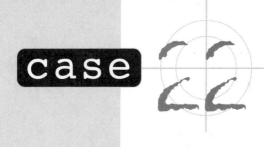

ID/CC A **40-year-old man** complains of **fever, cough, arthralgias,** and generalized malaise of 2 days' duration.

HPI He also complains of left-sided pleuritic chest pain and mentions that he recently noticed a few **painful red lesions** on his shins. Three days ago he returned from a trip to the **southwestern United States.**

PE VS: fever (38.9°C); tachypnea. PE: rales heard over left lower lobe; multiple tender **erythematous nodules** over both shins (ERYTHEMA NODOSUM); movements at large joints (knees and ankles) restricted by pain.

Labs CBC/PBS: eosinophilia; **coccidioidin skin test positive** (5-mm area of induration 48 hours after intradermal injection of coccidioidin).

Imaging CXR: right upper lobe infiltrate with hilar and paratracheal adenopathy.

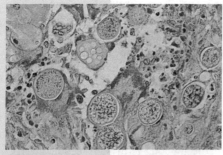

Figure 22-1. Spherules containing multiple endospores seen on tissue biopsy.

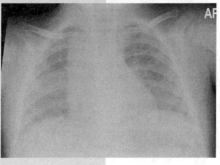

Figure 22-2. CXR: right upper lobe infiltrate with hilar and paratracheal adenopathy.

INFECTIOUS DISEASE

case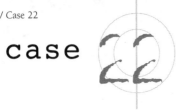

Coccidioidomycosis

Pathogenesis	The causative agent is *Coccidioides immitis*, a dimorphic fungus that grows in its natural soil habitat and on routine culture as a mold composed of **septate hyphae–bearing arthrospores**. The arthrospores are detached and swept into an aerosol that can easily be inhaled. Within the host, the highly infectious arthrospores mature into **spherules, the definitive tissue pathogen.** The spectrum of the disease varies from a primary pulmonary infection (whose severity varies from a mild influenza-like illness to severe pneumonitis) to a disseminated systemic form (more frequent in blacks and in pregnant or immunocompromised patients).
Epidemiology	The natural habitat of *C. immitis* is the desert soil of parts of California (eg, **San Joaquin Valley),** southern Arizona, Utah, New Mexico, Nevada, southwestern Texas, Mexico, and Central and South America. The recent increase in reported cases has been largely due to the increased prevalence of AIDS, recent dust storms and earthquakes, and increased physician recognition of the disease. **Human-to-human transmission does not occur.**
Management	Mild to moderate disease **usually resolves without treatment. Amphotericin B** is the treatment of choice for critically ill patients; follow with oral **itraconazole** or **ketoconazole** for long-term suppression in HIV-positive and immunocompromised patients. Surgery may be necessary for chronic and progressive pulmonary lesions.
Complications	Disseminated disease; chronic meningitis; skin lesions (maculopapular rash).
Breakout Point	

- Self-limited respiratory tract infection
- Occurs commonly in San Joaquin Valley (southern California)
- Occurs in farmers, archaeologists, and construction workers around soil

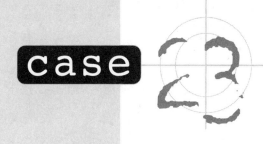

ID/CC A **35-year-old woman** presents with **delirium.**

HPI She suddenly developed an **influenza-like syndrome approximately 1 week ago.** It has included **fever, chills, headaches, rigors, malaise, and cough.** Over the past several days, she has also developed a **truncal rash** and has become less coherent.

PE VS: fever (38.7°C). PE: disoriented; prominent maculopapular rash on trunk with several incipient lesions on extremities; coarse breath sounds and rales bilaterally.

Labs CBC: elevated WBC; normal Hb, Hct, and platelets. **Weil-Felix test positive for antirickettsial antibodies.**

Imaging CXR: bilateral patchy pulmonary infiltrates.

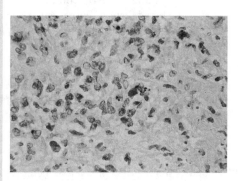

Figure 23-1. Intracellular location of rickettsia.

case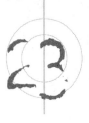

Epidemic Typhus

Pathogenesis

Epidemic typhus is caused by *Rickettsia prowazekii*, an obligate intracellular parasite that is **transmitted to humans by the body louse.** The disease begins when an infected individual is bitten by a louse, which ingests the rickettsial organism with the blood meal. The organism then multiplies in the gut of the louse. While biting another individual, the louse feces are excreted with *R. prowazekii*. The individual scratches, causing autoinoculation. One to three weeks after infection, the newly infected individual develops a flulike illness followed by a rash and signs of meningoencephalitis 5 to 9 days later.

Epidemiology

Epidemic typhus typically arises in times and places with **poor sanitation, crowding,** and **infrequent bathing.** Consequently, it has not been seen in the United States in more than 50 years. Among individuals who do contract the disease and are untreated, the mortality rate ranges from 10% to 60% and increases with age.

Management

Tetracycline (chloramphenicol second line). Prophylaxis depends on good **personal hygiene** and use of protective clothing in regions where typhus is prevalent. An inactivated vaccine of *R. prowazekii* is available abroad and for military personnel.

Complications

Myocarditis, intestinal hemorrhage, jaundice, renal insufficiency, vasculitis and thrombosis, and meningoencephalitis leading to delirium, coma, and death.

Breakout Point

- Epidemic typhus is a multiorgan vasculitis
- Occurs in Central and South America, Africa, and Asia (rare in United States)
- Prevalent in military personnel in endemic areas, with overcrowding and infrequent bathing
- Weil-Felix test detects antirickettsial antibodies
- Caused by *Rickettsia* and spread by the body louse (lice)

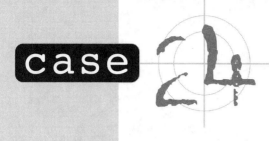

case 24

ID/CC	A **19-year-old male college student** complains of urinary urgency and **painful urination** (DYSURIA) for the past 3 days.
HPI	He also complains of painful **swelling of the left side of his scrotum** (due to epididymitis). He notes that his underwear has been stained with a **thick, greenish, purulent urethral discharge** that is more profuse in the morning. He had **unprotected sex** during spring break **1 week ago** with a local striptease dancer.
PE	VS: normal. PE: erythema and swelling of urethral meatus with a thick, greenish-yellow, purulent discharge expressed; **left epididymis swollen, hard, and exquisitely tender;** normal prostate.
Labs	CBC: leukocytosis (11,500); 75% neutrophils. Gram stain of urethral discharge shows **abundant PMNs** with **intracellular gram-negative diplococci;** culture in Thayer–Martin medium grows *Neisseria gonorrhoeae*; VDRL negative.
Imaging	None.

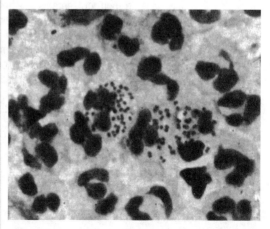

Figure 24-1. Gram stain of urethral discharge showing abundant PMNs with intracellular gram-negative diplococci.

case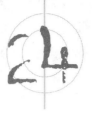

Gonorrhea

Pathogenesis

Gonorrhea is an STD caused by **Neisseria** *gonorrhoeae,* an oxidase-positive, **gram-negative, intracellular diplococcus.**

Epidemiology

Gonorrhea is a prevalent communicable disease in the United States. Its incubation period varies from 2 to 10 days; females are often asymptomatic carriers.

Management

Antibiotic therapy for uncomplicated disease consists of **ceftriaxone** (first line). Treatment should include **doxycycline** or azithromycin because of the possibility of coexisting infection with *Chlamydia trachomatis.* Complicated disease requires IV penicillin. Treatment of sexual partners is essential.

Complications

Patients may develop severe GU involvement and dissemination to virtually any organ or structure. Notable complications include PID with resultant sterility, septic monoarthritis, perihepatitis (FITZ–HUGH–CURTIS SYNDROME), and ophthalmia neonatorum in newborns.

Breakout Point

- Gram-negative intracellular diplococcus
- In men, presents as urethritis and penile discharge, can progress to epididymitis, orchitis, and unilateral scrotal pain
- In women, commonly is asymptomatic, or presents as vaginal discharge from cervicitis
- Can lead to PID, which can lead to ectopic pregnancy or sterility
- Empirically treat for both gonorrhea and *Chlamydia*

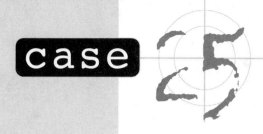

case

ID/CC	A **27-year-old sexually active man** presents with **painful penile lesions**.
HPI	The patient also complains of **burning, itching**, and a **tingling sensation**. The lesions have progressed from erythematous to vesicular to ulcerated.
PE	VS: low-grade fever (38.4°C). PE: numerous **vesicular and ulcerated lesions on** shaft of penis; inguinal lymphadenopathy.
Labs	Tzanck smear with multinucleated giant cells.
Imaging	None.

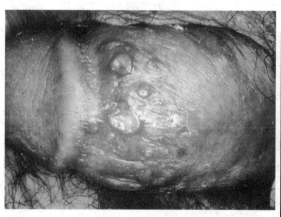

Figure 25-1. Numerous vesicular and ulcerated lesions on shaft of penis.

case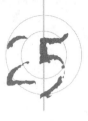

Herpes Genitalis

Pathogenesis | The causative agent is **HSV-2**; usually acquired and transmitted through sexual or perinatal contact. The virus replicates at the site of infection before migrating up neurons and becoming **latent in the sensory ganglia (trigeminal and lumbosacral)**; exposure to sunlight or UV light, immunosuppression, infections, fever, stress, hormonal changes, trauma, and depression may cause reactivation. HSV-2 causes genital herpes, neonatal herpes, and aseptic meningitis.

Epidemiology | One of the most common sexually transmitted infections.

Management | **Antiviral therapy** (eg, **acyclovir,** ganciclovir) for primary infections and to suppress genital recurrences. Foscarnet (IV) may be given for acyclovir-resistant cases or immunocompromised patients with systemic disease. Encourage prevention via latex condom use and cautious interpersonal contact with patients harboring active lesions.

Complications | HSV-1 is associated with encephalitis, herpetic whitlow (pustular lesion on the hand), esophagitis, and pneumonia. HSV-2 is associated with aseptic meningitis and neonatal herpes.

Breakout Point |
- Painful vesicles or ulcerative lesions on an erythematous base
- Positive Tzanck smear showing multinucleated giant cells and intranuclear inclusions
- Treated with acyclovir

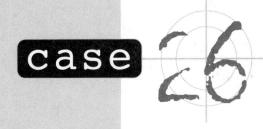
ID/CC A **72-year-old white man** presents with a **painful rash** on the right side of his chest.

HPI The patient has been taking medication for high blood pressure but is otherwise in excellent health. He also reports **severe burning pain preceding the appearance of the rash.**

PE VS: low-grade fever (38.1°C). PE: linear **dermatomal** distribution of painful vesicles on an erythematous base.

Labs Tzanck smear of vesicle base reveals large **multinucleated epithelial giant cells.**

Imaging None.

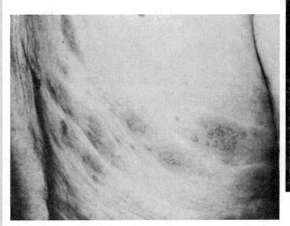

Figure 26-1. Linear **dermatomal** distribution of painful vesicles on an erythematous base.

INFECTIOUS DISEASE

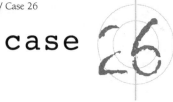

case

Herpes Zoster (Shingles)

Pathogenesis

The causative agent is **varialla zoster virus (VZV),** a double-stranded DNA virus of the herpesvirus family that causes two distinct pathologies: chickenpox (VARICELLA) and herpes zoster (SHINGLES). Chickenpox is a benign primary infection that is usually seen in children; herpes zoster results from **reactivation of the latent virus** and presents as a **dermatomal, painful vesicular rash.** When branches of the trigeminal nerve are involved, lesions may also appear in the mouth or tongue, around the eye (ZOSTER OPHTHALMICUS), and on the face. The precise mechanism of VZV reactivation is unknown, but it is thought that the virus remains latent in the dorsal root ganglion after a chickenpox infection; the dermatomes from T3 to L3 are most frequently involved.

Epidemiology

Herpes zoster can occur at all ages but primarily affects the elderly. Immunosuppressed patients are also at greater risk of more severe or disseminated infection.

Management

Analgesics for pain. **Antivirals** (eg, acyclovir), especially in zoster ophthalmicus, immunocompromised hosts, and **HIV-positive patients.** Give antibiotics for overlying skin infections; steroids may reduce inflammation and pain. **Zostavax** (VZV vaccine) is recommended for elderly patients.

Complications

Possible ophthalmic problems include conjunctivitis, keratitis, uveitis, and ocular muscle palsies; cerebral angiitis may result in focal neurologic deficits or ataxia. Other complications include postherpetic neuralgia and Ramsay Hunt syndrome. Disseminated disease may develop in immunocompromised patients (particularly lymphoma patients).

Breakout Point

- VZV causes chickenpox, which resolves; VZV can be reactivated later to cause herpes zoster (shingles)
- Vesicular rash along a single dermatome
- Postherpetic neuralgia can be extremely painful

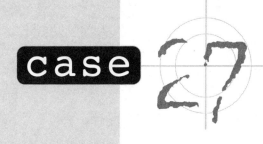

ID/CC A **40-year-old cave explorer** complains of chronic dry cough, malaise, weight loss, and night sweats.

HPI The patient is also a chronic **smoker** but has no history of hemoptysis and has not experienced significant shortness of breath. The patient states that he grew up in the **Ohio River valley** in the United States.

PE VS: **fever** (38.5°C). PE: scattered rales over both lung fields.

Labs CBC/PBS: anemia; leukopenia. Sputum culture: pending. Complement fixation test to check for specific titer: pending.

Imaging CXR: bronchopneumonia or multiple nodules are seen in primary form; apical fibronodular changes similar to TB in chronic form. XR, abdomen: calcification in the splenic area (seen in disseminated form).

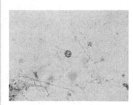

Figure 27-1. Mold form.

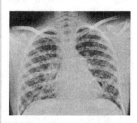

Figure 27-2. Disseminated disease showing diffuse interstitial alveolar infiltrates.

INFECTIOUS DISEASE

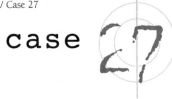

case 27

Histoplasmosis

Pathogenesis

The causative agent is *Histoplasma capsulatum*, a sporulating, dimorphic fungus that grows in soil (especially **soil enriched with the fecal material of chickens, starlings, and bats**); infection is acquired via **inhalation of spores** (due to aerosolization of fungus-laden soil). The organism has an affinity for fixed and circulating phagocytic cells of the reticuloendothelial system.

Epidemiology

Histoplasmosis is **endemic in the eastern-central United States;** the center of disease activity is the valleys of the Ohio and Mississippi Rivers. Although histoplasmosis has long been associated with farming and rural life, epidemic histoplasmosis has been increasingly reported among urban and suburban populations; the common denominator has been the disturbance of soil in and around a starling roost or accumulations of bat droppings.

Management

Most patients with primary pulmonary disease **do not require therapy.** Severely ill or immunocompromised patients and those with disseminated disease can be effectively treated with **amphotericin B** or **itraconazole.**

Complications

Disseminated histoplasmosis develops rarely. Clinical disseminated histoplasmosis may present as a systemic illness with multiple-organ system involvement that includes hepatosplenomegaly, generalized lymphadenopathy, fever, night sweats, anorexia, weight loss, anemia, and leukopenia. Adrenal insufficiency has been noted in 50% of these patients. In immunocompromised patients, progressive disseminated histoplasmosis is an important opportunistic infection. Chronic cavitary histoplasmosis affects middle-aged and elderly men who have severe COPD. Clinically, the disease is similar to cavitary TB.

Breakout Point

- Prevalent in the valleys of the Ohio and Mississippi Rivers
- Prevalent in chicken coop workers and cave explorers (bats)
- *H. capsulatum* is a dimorphic fungus (yeast or mold)
- Pulmonary macrophages in sputum are packed with multiple budding yeast organisms

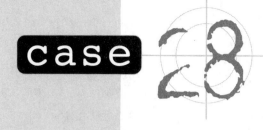

ID/CC A **15-year-old girl** complains of **malaise, fatigue,** and loss of appetite for the past week.

HPI She also complains of mild **fever** and **sore throat.** Her boyfriend recently experienced similar symptoms that lasted approximately 3 weeks.

PE VS: mild tachycardia; low-grade **fever** (38.2°C). PE: firm, discrete, tender, nonmatted cervical **lymphadenopathy** and **pharyngitis** with marked erythema and a diffuse exudate; **petechiae at junction of hard and soft palate;** no hepatomegaly but **mild soft splenomegaly.**

Labs CBC: leukocytosis with >50% lymphocytes and monocytes. PBS: >10% **atypical lymphocytes.** Monospot test for **heterophile antibodies positive;** specific EBV antibodies (EA, VLA, EBNA) also positive.

Imaging None.

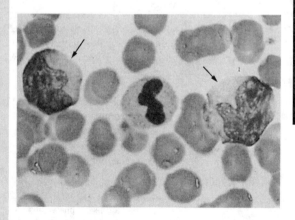

Figure 28-1. Peripheral blood smear: >10% atypical lymphocytes *arrows*.

case

Infectious Mononucleosis

Pathogenesis

Infectious mononucleosis is caused by **EBV**, a B-lymph-otrophic human herpesvirus; it is transmitted primarily by **salivary contact** (as in kissing) and shed intermittently by all seropositive (clinical and subclinical) individuals. Infectious mononucleosis is defined as the **triad of pharyngitis, fever, and lymphadenopathy combined with heterophile antibodies and atypical lymphocytosis**. A similar disease syndrome may be produced by other infections, such as toxoplasmosis, CMV, and HIV.

Epidemiology

Approximately 50% of the world's population has experienced a primary EBV infection before adolescence. Early infections are usually mild and subclinical, but a second wave of infection occurs at adolescence or adulthood that accounts for most cases of IM. The peak incidence of IM is 14 to 16 years for girls and 16 to 18 years for boys. EBV is associated with **nasopharyngeal carcinoma, Burkitt lymphoma**, certain types of **B-cell lymphomas** (especially in immunosuppressed individuals), and hairy leukoplakia in AIDS patients.

Management

Supportive care, adequate bed rest. **Glucocorticoids** may hasten the resolution of pharyngitis and are indicated for airway obstruction, severe thrombocytopenia, CNS involvement, or hemolytic anemia. **Acyclovir, ganciclovir**, and IVIG are potent inhibitors of EBV replication and halt oropharyngeal shedding; however, clinical benefits are minimal. **Avoid contact sports for 6 to 8 weeks because of the risk of splenic rupture.** Also avoid antibiotics, particularly ampicillin, because it may cause a skin rash that can be a diagnostic clue to EBV infections.

Complications

Complications include.

Breakout Point

- Triad of fever, pharyngitis, lymphadenopathy, with positive Monospot test (heterophile antibodies) and atypical lymphocytes
- Tender splenomegaly can lead to splenic rupture with trauma
- Treatment with ampicillin/amoxicillin can result in rash
- "Kissing disease" common in adolescents

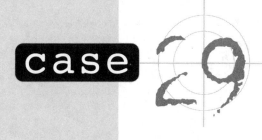

ID/CC A **76-year-old man** presents to the ER with **confusion** and a **severe cough**.

HPI The patient's illness began with the **abrupt onset of headache, muscle aches, and weakness** followed 24 hours later by **high fevers and shaking chills**. He subsequently developed a **nonproductive cough with pleuritic chest pain, dyspnea, nausea, vomiting**, and **diarrhea**. He is a chronic **smoker** and **drinks** heavily.

PE VS: **high fever** (40.0°C); **bradycardia** (HR 50); tachypnea; normal BP. PE: disoriented; diaphoretic; **crackles bilaterally.**

Labs CBC: **elevated WBC** (18,000). Lytes: **hyponatremia.** Gram stain of sputum reveals numerous neutrophils but no bacteria; **increased *Legionella* titers** by IFA. Culture on charcoal yeast extract medium positive for *Legionella*.

Imaging CXR: patchy bronchopneumonia.

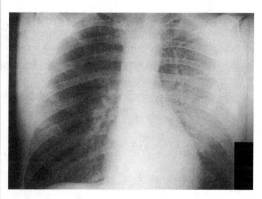

Figure 29-1. CXR: patchy bronchopneumonia

INFECTIOUS DISEASE

case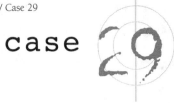

Legionella Pneumonia

Pathogenesis

Legionnaire disease is caused by **Legionella pneumo-phila**, a gram-negative aerobic bacillus that frequently resides in **environmental water sources;** acquired via **inhalation.** Infection is established in the presence of immunosuppression and/or impaired mucociliary clearance (as in smoking). Person-to-person transmission generally does not occur.

Epidemiology

Older age, smoking, and **depressed cell-mediated immunity** predispose to the development of this infection. The overall mortality rate is approximately 15%.

Management

Erythromycin is the drug of choice. Administer **rifampin in immunocompromised or severely ill patients.** Alternative antibiotics that may be effective include levofloxacin, azithromycin, and clarithromycin.

Complications

Dehydration, extrapulmonary infections, lung abscess, empyema, respiratory failure, pericarditis, endocarditis, myocarditis, shock, DIC, TTP, peritonitis, renal failure, pyelonephritis, and pancreatitis.

Breakout Point

- Associated with aerosolization/inhalation of contaminated water (air conditioners, humidifiers, whirlpool spas)
- Prevalent in elderly, immunocompromised patients
- Pneumonia that presents with abdominal pain and mental status change

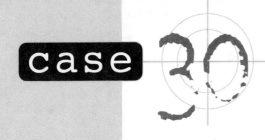

case

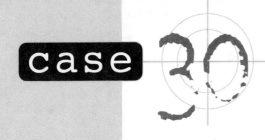

ID/CC A **22-year-old military recruit** presents with **altered mental status** following a bout of **high-grade fever.**

HPI Three days ago the patient had reported that he felt ill and complained of **headache, stiff neck,** a severe cough, a sore throat, chills, and muscle aches.

PE VS: **hypotension** (BP 82/40); **tachycardia** (HR 133); **fever** (39.6°C); tachypnea (RR 28). PE: **purpuric lesions** noted over axillae, flanks, wrists, and ankles; no papilledema.

Labs CBC: **leukopenia.** LP: CSF with low glucose, high protein, and many PMNs. **Gram-negative diplococci** on Gram stain; platelet count and circulating clotting factors decreased; blood culture yields **meningococci.**

Imaging None.

case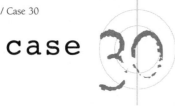

Meningococcemia

Pathogenesis

The causative agent is *Neisseria meningitidis*, a gram-negative diplococcus; spread by droplet infection and disseminated hematogenously from the nasopharynx. Produces the **Waterhouse–Friderichsen syndrome**, characterized by **meningitis, sepsis,** and **adrenal necrosis** (leading to fulminant vasomotor collapse and shock).

Epidemiology

Usually responsible for epidemic cases in the elderly population; however, any age group may be affected. A variable percentage of the population may carry the organism in the nasopharynx.

Management

Aggressive IV fluid and steroid replacement is key in vasomotor collapse secondary to adrenal failure. Administer cardiovascular or respiratory support as necessary. **Penicillin is the drug of choice** in meningococcal infection; third-generation cephalosporins (eg, ceftriaxone) may be given for empiric therapy, and chloramphenicol for β-lactam-allergic patients. Administer **rifampin prophylaxis for all household contacts.** Vaccination is recommended for immunodeficient or asplenic patients, those traveling to endemic areas, and military recruits.

Complications

Fulminant meningococcemia with shock, peripheral gangrene, DIC, acidosis, brain injury (due to meningitis), and long-term adrenal insufficiency.

Breakout Point

- Fever, positive Kernig and Brudzinski sign, altered mental status
- Rifampin prophylaxis is recommended for all household contacts
- Prevalent in military personnel and college students in dorms
- Complication is Waterhouse–Friderichsen syndrome (petechiae and shock)

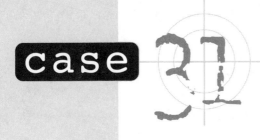

ID/CC A **58-year-old man** develops pleuritic chest pain, fever, and shaking chills.

HPI He also complains of a cough with **purulent sputum** formation. He is a chronic heavy **smoker with COPD.** He reports having had a **URI 1 week ago** with cough, coryza, and conjunctivitis.

PE VS: **high fever** (39.4°C); tachycardia (HR 117); tachypnea (RR 23); normal BP. PE: mild respiratory distress; **decreased breath sounds, inspiratory rales, dullness to percussion,** and **increased tactile fremitus** over right lower lung field.

Labs CBC: **leukocytosis** (17,500) with **neutrophilia** (84%). Elevated ESR. Lytes: normal. Sputum Gram stain shows **gram-positive diplococci in pairs** and many PMNs; sputum culture confirms *Streptococcus pneumoniae* (positive in only 25% of patients); blood cultures usually negative (positive in only 25% of patients).

Imaging CXR: lobar consolidation in the right upper lobe bounded inferiorly by the horizontal fissure.

INFECTIOUS DISEASE

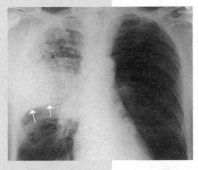

Figure 31-1. CXR: lobar consolidation in the right upper lobe bounded inferiorly by the horizontal fissure.

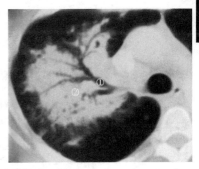

Figure 31-2. CT, chest: an air bronchogram (1) is seen in area of consolidation (2) (a different case).

61

case 31

Pneumococcal Pneumonia

Pathogenesis

S. pneumoniae lung infection is a major cause of **lobar pneumonia** and typically affects those who are at the **extremes of age** or those who have an underlying disease. For example, asplenic patients are unable to efficiently clear nonopsonized bacteria from the blood.

Epidemiology

Pneumococcal pneumonia usually follows a URI and is more common in patients with chronic cardiopulmonary disease as well as in sickle cell disease and asplenic (or splenectomized) patients, in whom disease is more severe. It is also more common among smokers, renal failure patients, alcoholics, and immunocompromised patients (HIV). There is a higher incidence in late winter and early spring.

Management

Hospitalize if the patient is older than 65 years of age and has concurrent illnesses, is severely ill, or is homeless. Start empiric antibiotics based on the likely pathogen. **Pneumococcus** is the most common cause of CAP; **penicillin** is the textbook drug of choice. Ceftriaxone, vancomycin, or fluoroquinolones may be effective for the treatment of penicillin-resistant pneumococcal infections. For atypical pneumonia, *Mycoplasma* and *Chlamydia* are common pathogens; a macrolide is the drug of choice. For CAP requiring hospitalization, also consider *Haemophilus influenzae*, gram-negative rods, and *Legionella* as the cause; give second- or third-generation cephalosporin. For nosocomial pneumonia, consider *Pseudomonas, Staphylococcus aureus, Escherichia coli,* and *Klebsiella* as the cause; give empiric therapy with third-generation cephalosporin and aminoglycoside. Prevent with pneumococcal vaccine for patients who undergo splenectomy as well as those who have malignancies, sickle cell disease, or COPD.

Complications

Atelectasis, bacteremia, meningitis, parapneumonic pleural effusion, lung abscess, pericarditis, and empyema.

Breakout Point

- Three most common causes of typical CAP:
  S. pneumoniae, H. influenzae, Moraxella catarrhalis
- Characterized by fever, cough, sputum production, rales, tactile fremitus, and E to A change
- Air bronchograms on chest imaging

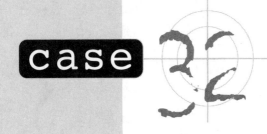

case

ID/CC A **23-year-old woman** complains of the appearance of a **prominent diffuse rash** over the past 2 to 3 days.

HPI The patient adds that about **1 week** before the rash appeared, she felt tired and had a **low-grade fever**; swollen cheeks and lymph nodes; mild nasal congestion; itchy eyes; and minor **joint aches** in her fingers, wrists, and knees. The rash **started on her face, spread to her trunk, and then spread down her arms and legs,** with each phase lasting about 1 day. She denies any sexual activity and denies the possibility of pregnancy.

PE VS: normal. PE: **diffuse maculopapular rash; petechial exanthem on soft palate** (FORSCHHEIMER SPOTS) noted along with **patchy erythema** in oropharynx without exudate; mild nasal erythema without exudate; soft, movable **lymphadenopathy** noted in **postauricular** and posterior cervical distribution.

Labs ELISA demonstrates **rubella-specific IgM and IgG antibodies** (acute rubella shows fourfold or higher increase in IgG titer). CBC: thrombocytopenia. Pregnancy test negative.

Imaging None.

case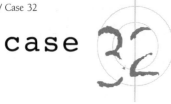

Rubella (German Measles)

Pathogenesis

The causative agent is rubella virus, a **togavirus**. Transmission is via droplets shed in respiratory secretions, infecting the respiratory tract and, subsequently, the bloodstream, resulting in the characteristic rash, fever, and lymphadenopathy.

Epidemiology

Due to greater than 95% seroconversion of vaccinated individuals, routine use of the live attenuated vaccine has virtually eliminated epidemic outbreaks of rubella among school-age children; **most cases now occur in young adults.** Although it is often subclinical, rubella is highly contagious, albeit less so than measles; it is transmissible via **respiratory droplets** from 1 week prior to the appearance of the rash to 15 days afterward, with the incubation period ranging from 14 to 21 days (average 18 days). Natural infection leads to lifelong immunity; antibody to rubella crosses the placenta and thereby protects the newborn.

Management

There is **no specific therapy** for rubella; the management of acute rubella consists of the **symptomatic relief** of fever (acetaminophen), arthralgias, arthritis, encephalitis, thrombocytopenia, and so on. All infants should be **immunized with live attenuated virus vaccine** (the **first dose administered between 12 and 15 months of age** and **another dose given during childhood**). **Pregnant women should not be immunized,** and birth control should be practiced for a minimum of 3 months following vaccine administration. Consider therapeutic abortion if exposure occurs during pregnancy. **No serious side effects** have been reported after the administration of rubella **vaccine to immunocompromised** individuals.

Complications

Congenital abnormalities, which include early-onset cataracts, glaucoma, microphthalmia, hearing deficits, heart defects, and psychomotor retardation, occur primarily if the fetus is infected during the first trimester. Rarely, patients (adults more commonly than children) develop postinfectious encephalopathy that begins 1 to 6 days after the appearance of the rash.

Breakout Point

- "3-day measles"
- Prodromal symptoms few days before rash
- Pink maculopapular rash (exanthem) starting on face/neck and spreads centrifugally to trunk and extremities in 1 day

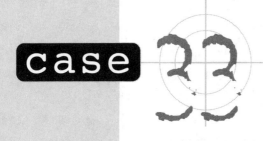

case 33

ID/CC A **30-year-old man** presents to the dermatology out-patient clinic complaining of a **generalized rash** and **hair loss**.

HPI The skin eruption is nonpruritic. He reports having had **unprotected sexual intercourse** with multiple partners; on directed questioning he notes that he had a **painless ulcer** (CHANCRE) on his penis a few weeks ago.

PE **Maculopapular skin rash** over entire body, including **palms and soles**; patches of hair loss involving scalp and eyebrows (FOLLICULAR SYPHILIDES); generalized nontender lymphadenopathy; mucous patches (silver-gray erosions with a red periphery) seen on tongue; **condylomata lata** (broad, moist, gray-white lesions) seen in perianal and intertriginous groin area; edges of skin are indurated (ELLIOT SIGN).

Labs Darkfield examination of specimens obtained from condylomata and mucous patches reveals presence of treponemes; RPR positive; **VDRL titers increased** (>1:32); FTA-ABS test (confirmatory) positive.

Imaging None.

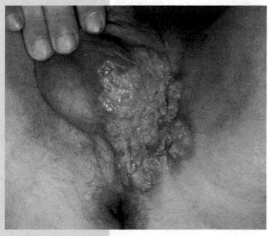

Figure 33-1.
Condylomata lata (moist, gray-white lesions) in groin area.

65

INFECTIOUS DISEASE

case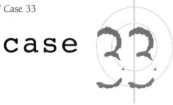

Syphilis: Secondary

Pathogenesis

Causative agent is *Treponema pallidum*. Usually transmitted during sexual activity by direct contact with the mucocutaneous lesions that arise during the primary or secondary stage of syphilis (tertiary syphilis is rarely transmissible); however, vertical transmission from an untreated pregnant woman (maximum risk during 16 to 36 weeks' gestation) may result in congenital syphilis in the fetus.

Epidemiology

In the United States, the incidence of syphilis diminished markedly from the 1940s through the 1970s as a result of the introduction of antibiotics. Since then there have been two epidemics in the United States; the first, which occurred in the early 1980s and primarily involved homosexual and bisexual males, subsequently declined due to sexual behavior modification among this group in response to the risk of AIDS. The second epidemic, which occurred during the second half of the 1980s, primarily involved women, adolescents, and heterosexuals who exchanged sex for drugs or money. Approximately **one-half** of those involved in sexual activity with individuals infected with syphilis become infected.

Management

Benzathine penicillin G administered intramuscularly; if patient is sensitive to penicillin, erythromycin or doxycycline can be used. **Follow up with VDRL levels.** The CSF should be examined if the VDRL titer does not become negative or does not decrease dramatically in 6 months; if the CSF is abnormal, treat as for neurosyphilis. If relapse develops, patients should also be tested for HIV infection.

Complications

Tertiary syphilis, which includes neurosyphilis, Argyll Robertson pupil abnormalities (afferent pupil defect), tabes dorsalis (destruction of posterior spinal columns), and syphilitic aortitis.

Breakout Point

- Primary syphilis: genital chancre
- Secondary syphilis: rash on palms and soles, condyloma lata
- Tertiary syphilis: gummas, syphilitic aortitis, neurosyphilis

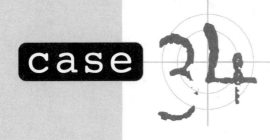

case

ID/CC	A **45-year-old man** with a history of **untreated vene-real disease** complains of **pain in his legs** and **difficulty walking,** especially in the dark.
HPI	For the past year, the patient has noted sporadic episodes of electric-like **"lightning" pain in his legs** that lasts for hours or days. He also complains of persistent numbness and tingling (feeling of "pins and needles") in his feet and has been **"stumbling"** whenever he turns quickly.
PE	VS: normal. PE: **discrepancy in pupillary size** (ANISOCORIA); involved pupil **reacts poorly to light but normally to accommodation** (ARGYLL ROBERTSON PUPIL); cranial nerves grossly intact; motor exam 5/5 bilaterally throughout; DTRs 2+ and symmetric in upper extremities but **absent at patella and Achilles;** Babinski absent bilaterally; sensory exam reveals **decreased vibratory and proprioception sense** in feet; **Romberg sign positive;** patient maintains knees in an extended position; finger-to-nose intact bilaterally (tests cerebellar function).
Labs	CBC/Lytes: normal. PT/PTT and glucose normal; **serum FTA-ABS positive.** LP: **lymphocytic pleocytosis;** protein of 80 mg/dL; normal glucose; **positive FTA-ABS; positive oligoclonal bands** (FTA-ABS test is more sensitive and specific for the detection of treponemal antigens than VDRL).
Imaging	None.

INFECTIOUS DISEASE

case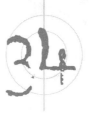

Neurosyphilis (Tabes Dorsalis)

Pathogenesis

Tabes dorsalis is a form of **neurosyphilis** that is characterized by **chronic progressive demyelination** of the posterior column of the spinal cord, posterior sensory ganglia (dorsal root ganglia), and nerve roots. *Treponema pallidum*, a spirochete, is the causative organism; it usually invades the CNS 3 to 18 months after systemic infection occurs.

Epidemiology

The incidence of latent syphilis is 7.4 per 100,000 in the United States.

Management

Treat with **IV penicillin.** If the patient is allergic to penicillin, he should undergo desensitization and then proceed with penicillin. Follow response to therapy by checking LP repeatedly over 2 years. Expect normalization of CSF VDRL by 1 year; relapse after 2 years of negative CSF is uncommon.

Complications

Complications include **Charcot joints** (joint damage due to decreased sensation of lower limbs), incontinence secondary to neurogenic bladder, painless ulcers over pressure points, hearing loss, and visual loss due to uveitis, chorioretinitis, or optic neuritis. **Tabes crises** consist of abdominal pain and bladder dysfunction.

Breakout Point

- Tabes dorsalis, Argyll Robertson pupil, tertiary syphilis
- Difficulty walking in the dark and wide-based gait (proprioception)
- Loss of vibratory sense
- Can present as severe abdominal pain with vomiting or lightning pains in legs

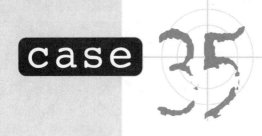

ID/CC	A **35-year-old HIV-positive man** complains of increasing fatigue, weight loss, fever, and a progressively worsening cough of 6 weeks' duration.
HPI	He also acknowledges having **frequent night sweats.** He has no known TB contacts but is known to have had **HIV infection** for 3 years; his last CD4 count was 150.
PE	VS: fever (39.5°C). PE: thin, lethargic; oral thrush; mild cervical lymphadenopathy bilaterally; mild rales audible in bilateral apices.
Labs	Sputum cultures positive for **acid-fast bacilli**; PPD and anergy panel nonreactive (secondary to immunosuppression); cultures eventually grow *Mycobacterium tuberculosis*.
Imaging	CXR: primary complex with ill-defined right upper lobe consolidation.

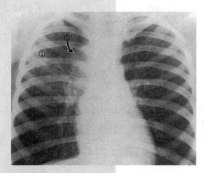

Figure 35-1. CXR: primary complex with ill-defined right upper lobe consolidation (1) and right paratracheal adenopathy (2 and arrow).

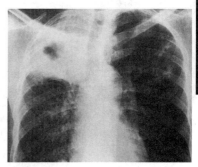

Figure 35-2. CXR: postprimary TB with right upper lobe consolidation and central cavitation.

case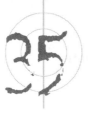

Tuberculosis: Pulmonary

Pathogenesis

The causative agent is *M. tuberculosis*; infection is acquired **via inhalation of aerosolized droplets** that reach the lungs. Bacteria are then ingested by macrophages and are killed or persist and multiply. Organisms may disseminate to the lymphatic system and bloodstream until they are walled off by granulomatous inflammation (due to **type IV hypersensitivity reaction**). This process of primary infection is typically asymptomatic. Viable organisms remain dormant for years and may reactivate disease when host defenses are compromised.

Epidemiology

The incidence of TB continues to increase worldwide. The frequency of atypical presentations also continues to increase, particularly in the **elderly,** patients with **HIV** infection, and nursing home residents. HIV infection represents the most important risk factor for TB today; the recent increase in the incidence of TB can be attributed to the HIV epidemic. Multidrug-resistant strains of *M. tuberculosis* are now seen with increasing frequency.

Management

Immediate respiratory isolation. Start treatment with a **four-drug regimen of INH, rifampin, pyrazinamide,** and **ethambutol.** Directly observed therapy is an option for noncompliant patients. A presumptive diagnosis requires acid-fast bacilli on smear or a positive PPD in patients with CXR findings. A culture is required to confirm the diagnosis and to narrow antimycobacterial coverage. Five- or six-drug regimens should be used for outbreaks of strains resistant to INH and rifampin. Give supplemental **oral pyridoxine,** which prevents neuropathy due to vitamin B_6 deficiency caused by INH. **Chemoprophylaxis** with INH or rifampin for 12 months should be given to high-risk individuals, close contacts of patients with INH-resistant TB, patients with positive tuberculin skin tests (<35 years of age), and any of the following: known or suspected HIV infection, close contacts of newly diagnosed patients, recent converters, and patients with chronic illness. Immunization with BCG (results in a positive PPD) is widely used in developing countries where the incidence of TB is high but is not used in the United States at this time.

Complications

Lobar or segmental collapse or consolidation, pleural effusion, pericardial involvement, tuberculoma formation, meningitis, and miliary TB.

Breakout Point

- Induration, not erythema, 48–72 hours after PPD
- HIV-positive status, abnormal CXR, recent known TB contact: 5 mm induration
- Nursing home/shelter residents, prisoners, IV drug use, or reception of BCG at birth: 10 mm induration
- Normal (young and in good health): 15 mm induration

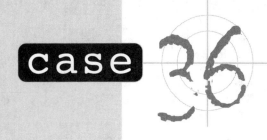

case 36

ID/CC   A **24-year-old man** complains of **persistent fever** of 2 weeks' duration along with mild **abdominal pain, constipation, a skin rash**, and a sore throat and cough.

HPI   He additionally complains of malaise, myalgias, arthralgias, and headaches. He reports having traveled to Mexico recently, where he ate **food** from **street vendors.**

PE   VS: **bradycardia** (HR 50); **fever** (38.5°C); normal BP. PE: confluent macular **erythematous rash on the trunk** that fades on pressure (ROSE SPOTS); abdomen mildly distended and tender but with no peritoneal signs; mild **hepatosplenomegaly.**

Labs   CBC: anemia; **neutropenia.** Widal test reveals **elevated "O" antigen titer** of 1:320 (>1:160 is diagnostic); blood and stool cultures positive for *Salmonella typhi.* UA: proteinuria; various casts.

Imaging   CXR: normal (may show free subdiaphragmatic air in typhoid intestinal perforation).

INFECTIOUS DISEASE

case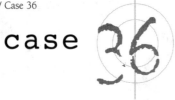

Typhoid Fever

Pathogenesis

The causative agent is *Salmonella typhi*. Typhoid fever predominantly affects human lymphoid tissue; the incubation period is variable (3 to 60 days) and is inversely proportional to the number of bacilli ingested. Infection classically results in **longitudinal ulcers in the ileum** (along Peyer patches) and perforation (typically after 3 weeks of the disease), with subsequent peritonitis and variable patterns of GI bleeding leading to hypotension and hypovolemic shock.

Epidemiology

Typhoid fever has a worldwide distribution but is predominantly a disease of **developing countries** (due to poor sanitation). It is transmitted through **contaminated food or drink** (starchy foods, shellfish, eggs, and beverages, including milk); through **contact with the feces or urine** of patients or asymptomatic carriers (females with typhoid cholecystitis and patients with *Schistosoma hematobium* urine infections are frequently carriers); and by **houseflies,** which may act as mechanical vectors. Typhoid fever is associated with significant morbidity and mortality, approaching 15%.

Management

The primary antibiotic choices include **ceftriaxone** or **ciprofloxacin.** If the patient is in shock, administer **dexamethasone** before antibiotics. In the event of treatment failure or perforation, **laparotomy with resection** of the affected segment is indicated. Fluoroquinolones are contraindicated in children and pregnant women. Asymptomatic carriers may require cholecystectomy if they fail antibiotic therapy. Prevention involves hygienic/dietary measures; **typhoid vaccine** is advised for those traveling to endemic areas.

Complications

Septic shock, intestinal perforation and bleeding, endocarditis, pneumonia, cholecystitis, and meningitis.

Breakout Point

- Caused by *Salmonella typhi*
- Can cause a "rose spot" rash, "green pea soup" diarrhea

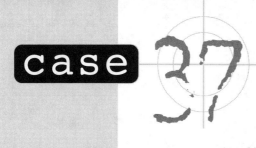

case 37

ID/CC   A **50-year-old woman** presents after suffering a **tonic-clonic seizure.**

HPI   She also complains of weakness in the right arm and leg and has been experiencing a severe **headache, projectile vomiting,** and **blurring of vision.** She has traveled to **Mexico** within the past 5 years.

PE   VS: normal. PE: **papilledema;** motor weakness with increased tone noted in right arm and leg; DTRs exaggerated on right side; plantar response on right side is extensor; multiple nontender subcutaneous nodules noted over abdomen, arms, and neck.

Labs   CBC: eosinophilia. **Serum serology for cysticercosis positive.** LP (performed once elevated ICP is lowered): mononuclear cell-predominant pleocytosis; elevated proteins; low glucose.

Imaging   MR/CT, head: **multiple ring-enhancing lesions** involving the left cortex surrounded by considerable edema. XR, arm: multiple small soft tissue calcifications known as "puffed rice" lesions.

INFECTIOUS DISEASE

case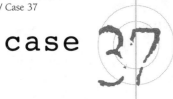

Cysticercosis

Pathogenesis

The causative agent of cysticercosis is *Taenia solium.* **Intestinal infection** occurs through the **ingestion of undercooked pork containing cysticerci.** Ingestion of *T. solium* eggs may also occur through consumption of **food contaminated** by egg-containing feces or by **autoinfection** involving hand-to-mouth fecal carriage. Clinical presentation depends on the organ compromised by the cysticerci; the most serious forms of cysticercosis are those with **ocular, cardiac,** and **neurologic** involvement.

Epidemiology

Most infections are encountered in **developing countries,** where intestinal *T. solium* infections occur frequently. In endemic regions, cysticercosis is the most common cause of seizure disorders.

Management

Praziquantel and **albendazole** are the mainstays of therapy. Give **corticosteroids** to limit inflammatory reactions to dying cysticerci; these reactions render ocular and spinal cysticercosis untreatable. CT scans should be repeated 3 to 6 months after therapy to evaluate cyst viability, and therapy should be repeated if viable cysts remain.

Complications

Seizures, hydrocephalus, and chronic meningitis.

Breakout Point

- From undercooked pork
- Multiple ring-enhancing lesions in brain
- Treat with praziquantel or albendazole

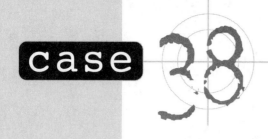

case

ID/CC A **32-year-old man** is brought to the ER with **headache**, nausea, vomiting, and **fever.**

HPI The patient is a former **IV drug user** who also complains of cough and shortness of breath. His next-door neighbor raises **pigeons** as a hobby.

PE VS: **low-grade fever** (38.5°C); tachycardia (HR 146); hypotension (BP 80/55). PE: **altered sensorium; mild nuchal rigidity; papilledema;** oral thrush.

Labs CBC: anemia; lymphopenia; decreased CD4+ T-cell count. LP: CSF with **lymphocytic pleocytosis,** increased protein, and decreased glucose. **India ink** preparation demonstrates round, yeastlike cells; **latex agglutination test for cryptococcal antigen positive;** HIV ELISA positive.

Imaging CXR: lobar disease, pleural effusion, and hilar adenopathy. MR, brain: cerebral atrophy; no communicating hydrocephalus; **scattered focal** lesions.

INFECTIOUS DISEASE

case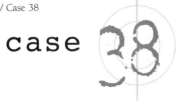

Meningitis: Cryptococcal

Pathogenesis

The causative agent is *Cryptococcus neoformans*. The **most common opportunistic systemic fungal infection in patients with AIDS,** cryptococcosis is acquired via the respiratory route and disseminated hematogenously to the CNS. It most commonly affects the **meninges.**

Epidemiology

In the United States, half of all cases of cryptococcosis are found in **AIDS patients;** of those patients who are not HIV positive, most are **immunosuppressed. Pigeon droppings** and eucalyptus trees are considered significant environmental reservoirs.

Management

IV amphotericin B with **flucytosine; fluconazole** for maintenance therapy. Begin fluconazole after the CD4+ count drops below 100 cells/μL for candidal and cryptococcal prophylaxis.

Complications

With advancing illness, brainstem compression, coma, and death may occur rapidly. Pulmonary cryptococcosis may manifest as chest pain and cough; skin and osteolytic bone lesions may occur. Rarely, hepatitis, endophthalmitis, pericarditis, and endocarditis may occur. Acute renal failure may occur with amphotericin B.

Breakout Point

- India ink prep shows capsule around yeast
- Prevalent in patients with AIDS
- *C. neoformans* found in pigeon droppings

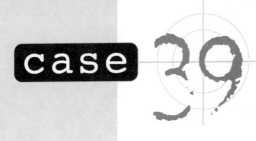
ID/CC A **36-year-old man** presents to the ER complaining of sudden-onset **pain and swelling in his knee** of 3 hours' duration.

HPI The patient is a basketball player who reports having had **repeated arthroscopic procedures** on both knees. In addition to his sudden pain, he notes associated **fever and chills**. No other joint involvement was noted, and he denies any prior heart valve disease or IV drug use.

PE VS: fever (39.4°C). PE: back, hip, and ankle exams normal. Left knee shows significant **induration, erythema, warmth, and marked tenderness to light palpation**; active range of motion limited by pain; passive range of motion intact; drawer tests negative.

Labs CBC: **marked leukocytosis** (>100,000 with >90% PMNs). Synovial fluid analysis shows **pleocytosis** (>100,000 with >90% PMNs) and **low glucose**; Gram stain positive for gram-positive cocci in clusters; culture reveals *Staphylococcus aureus*.

Imaging XR, knee: normal (normal early, but may manifest demineralization within a few days; complicating features such as osteomyelitis or periostitis may be seen as bony erosions or joint space narrowing within 2 weeks).

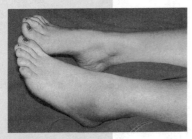

Figure 39-1. Edema and erythema of the left ankle.

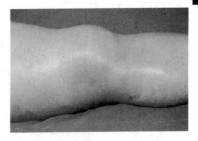

Figure 39-2. Left knee shows significant induration, erythema, warmth, and marked tenderness to light palpation

case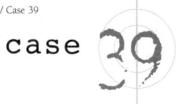

Septic Arthritis: Staphylococcal

Pathogenesis

Septic arthritis is characterized by **acute bacterial infection of a joint.** Etiologically, it is classified as either **gonococcal** (causative agent, *Neisseria gonorrhoeae*) or **nongonococcal** (most common causative agent, *Staphylococcus aureus*). Bacteria enter the affected joint via the **bloodstream,** having spread from a **neighboring site of infection** (eg, bone or soft tissue), or by **direct inoculation.** Gonococcal arthritis, which accounts for up to half of all cases, is distinguished by prodromal migratory polyarthralgias, tenosynovitis, purulent monoarthritis, and a characteristic maculopapular or vesicular rash. Patients may or may not have accompanying GU complaints. Nongonococcal acute bacterial arthritis presents with sudden-onset monoarticular arthritis in weight-bearing joints with large joint effusions and occurs almost exclusively in individuals with known predisposing factors. Infections involving *S. aureus* usually arise after **surgery, penetrating injury,** or **other predisposing factors.**

Epidemiology

Predisposing factors include **damaged joints** (osteoarthritis, RA, trauma, repeated procedures or surgeries), **persistent septicemia** (IV drug use, endocarditis), **immunosuppression** (malignancy, HIV, end-stage renal disease), and **prosthetic joints** (loss of normal local host defenses).

Management

Administration of **IV penicillinase-resistant β-lactam antibiotics** in combination with third-generation cephalosporin (eg, cefotaxime or ceftriaxone) provides coverage for most infections. Local measures include hot compresses, joint immobilization (splint/traction), rest, and elevation. The drug of choice for gonococcal arthritis (based on joint aspirate Gram stain) is IV ceftriaxone. Gonococcal arthritis responds promptly to antibiotic therapy within 24 to 48 hours, leading to complete recovery in nearly all cases. Nongonococcal arthritis also responds rapidly to antibiotic therapy in the absence of severe underlying disease. **Local aspiration** may be required with persistent reaccumulation of effusions. **Surgical drainage** is indicated with hip involvement (poor access by aspiration) or when medical therapy fails.

Complications

Delayed or inadequate treatment may result in permanent articular destruction and bony ankylosis.

Breakout Point

- Joint edema, erythema, warmth, tenderness with effusion
- WBC >50,000–100,000
- History of joint disease, surgery, or penetrating trauma

case 40

ID/CC A **19-year-old man** on his first postoperative day after splenectomy experiences **marked oliguria** (<20 mL urine/hr) and complains of **malaise, anorexia, and nausea.**

HPI He was found in **shock** after having been in a motorcycle accident. An immediate laparotomy was performed after rehydration, and a ruptured spleen with a **large hemoperitoneum** was found.

PE VS: normal. PE: well hydrated; **no suprapubic mass** palpable (enlargement of bladder in cases of postrenal ARF).

Labs CBC: anemia; **leukocytosis with left shift. Increased BUN and creatinine (BUN/creatinine ratio 10:20). Lytes: hyperkalemia; hyperphosphatemia.** ABGs: **metabolic acidosis.** UA: proteinuria; **renal tubular cell and granular casts;** urine specific gravity 1.012; urinary osmolality <350 mOsm/kg; Fe_{Na} >1%; urine sodium >20 mEq/L.

Imaging US, renal: no ureteral dilatation or enlargement of the kidney.

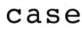

case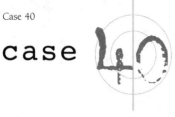

Acute Tubular Necrosis: Ischemic

Pathogenesis

ARF may be oliguric (<30 mL/h) or nonoliguric and is classically divided into prerenal, intrinsic renal, and postrenal. **Prerenal ARF** is caused by a decrease in effective extracellular volume with decreased renal perfusion; it is associated with prolonged vomiting and diarrhea, acute blood loss (traumatic, GI, or gynecologic bleeding), fluid retention with heart disease (CHF), cirrhosis, drugs (NSAIDs, ACE inhibitors), vascular contraction, diuretics, and fluid sequestration (eg, from pancreatitis, burns, peritonitis). Laboratory tests show muddy brown or hyaline casts, a BUN/creatinine ratio >20, urine sodium <10 mEq/L, Fe_{Na} <1%, urine osmolality >500 mOsm/kg, and urine specific gravity >1.018. **Renal** (INTRINSIC) **failure** is caused by prolonged ischemia (the most common cause of ATN, as in this case), nephrotoxins (cisplatin, **contrast media, aminoglycosides**), and diffuse renal cortical necrosis. **Postrenal** causes of ARF include any **obstruction to urine flow** from the kidney to the urethra, such as kidney stones, pelvic surgery, bladder or prostate tumors, retroperitoneal fibrosis, pelvic tumors, and urethral stricture.

Management

Insert a **Foley catheter** and measure postvoid volume to rule out obstruction. If the patient is volume depleted, administer isotonic saline solution and wait for diuresis; if euvolemic, administer furosemide or dopamine. **Correct acidosis and electrolyte abnormalities** (hyperkalemia, hyperphosphatemia). Adjust medications according to creatinine clearance. **Dialysis** is indicated in severe hyperkalemia, pulmonary edema, refractory acidosis, fluid overload, pericarditis, and uremic encephalopathy.

Complications

Complications include encephalopathy, GI bleeding (impaired platelet function), salt and fluid overload, pericarditis, severe hyperkalemia, hypocalcemia, increased anion-gap metabolic acidosis, and anemia. Opportunistic infections, poor wound healing, and muscle wasting occur due to the hypercatabolic state that is related to uremia and infection.

Breakout Point

- Prerenal: hypovolemia, CHF, shock, drugs causing vasoconstriction (NSAIDs, ACE inhibitors)
- Intrarenal: intrinsic renal disease, atheroembolic renal disease, malignant hypertension
- Postrenal: obstructive uropathy (benign prostatic hyperplasia)

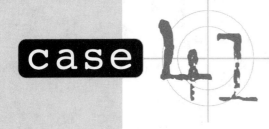

case 41

ID/CC A **55-year-old woman** with gram-negative septicemia becomes lethargic and develops **decreased urine output.**

HPI The patient was started on **IV gentamicin** 3 days ago. She subsequently developed increasing **confusion.**

PE VS: low-grade fever (38.7°C); tachycardia (HR 110); tachypnea; hypotension (BP 90/50). PE: **disoriented; pericardial rub; asterixis.**

Labs Lytes: elevated potassium and phosphate. Elevated BUN and creatinine; blood cultures reveal gram-negative bacilli. UA: proteinuria; muddy brown casts with renal tubular epithelial casts in sediment; decreased urinary osmolality (<300 mOsm/kg); specific gravity 1.012; Fe_{Na} >1%. ABGs: metabolic acidosis.

Imaging None.

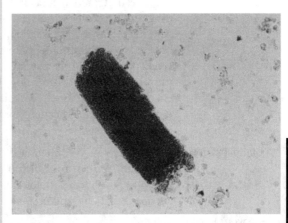

Figure 41-1. Muddy brown casts with renal tubular epithelial casts in sediment.

case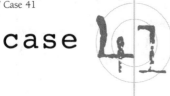

Acute Tubular Necrosis: Toxic

Pathogenesis

ATN occurs secondary to an **ischemic or nephrotoxic insult,** causing focal tubular epithelial cell necrosis leading to **preglomerular vasoconstriction, tubular obstruction** by necrotic tubular epithelial cells and formed casts, and **tubular back leak.** Consequently, tubular flow decreases and intratubular pressure increases, yielding a lower GFR and ultimately oliguria. Oliguria results in **salt and water retention, hyperkalemia, uremia**, and a **metabolic acidosis.**

Epidemiology

ATN is the **most frequent cause of acute renal failure.** Risk factors are classified as **toxic** (radiographic contrast, antibiotics, heavy metals, organic solvents, hemoglobinuria, myoglobinuria) or **ischemic** (decreased cardiac output, hemorrhage, sepsis).

Management

Correct the underlying etiology; monitor fluid balance; restrict protein intake; discontinue offending drugs; and correct electrolytes. If hypovolemia exists without evidence of obstruction, volume should be repleted to **maintain adequate cardiac output and renal perfusion.** After patients are euvolemic, start **diuretics** to promote urine flow. Uremic pericarditis, encephalopathy, severe hyperkalemia, and overt volume overload are indications for **peritoneal dialysis** or **hemodialysis.**

Complications

Renal failure in ATN often lasts 10 to 20 days, with **complete return to normal** renal functioning. Complications include fluid retention, hyperkalemia, anemia, infections, and uremia.

Breakout Point

- History of an ischemic or toxic event
- Muddy brown casts in urine
- Acute renal failure that is reversible

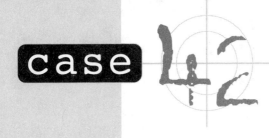

case 42

ID/CC A 65-year-old man presents with mildly foamy urine and fatigue, which he has had for the past month.

HPI He has had **type 2 DM for the past 30 years.** Urine microalbumin has been persistently high over the past 5 years. His blood glucose readings are generally 200–300 at home, and his Hb A1c has always been high. He was diagnosed with diabetic retinopathy 2 years ago.

PE VS: **hypertensive**. PE: well-appearing, obese; OD 20/150, OU 20/100; normal pupillary reflex; mild pitting edema throughout; decreased sensation to pinprick and decreased reflexes in lower extremities; decreased dorsopedal pulses.

Labs UA: protein >400 mg/dL (>3 g/day), 3+ glucose, microalbumin high. CBC: anemic. Chem 7: mildly elevated BUN and creatinine.

Imaging US, kidneys: mildly enlarged kidneys bilaterally. EM: dramatic thickening of GBMs.

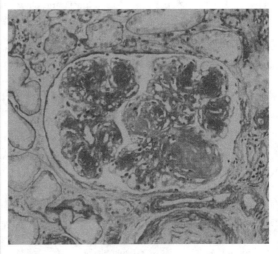

Figure 42-1. Diffuse and nodular glomerulosclerosis with Kimmelstiel-Wilson nodules.

case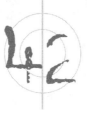

Diabetic Nephropathy

Pathogenesis

Accumulation of **advanced glycation end products (AGEs)** leads to crosslinking and **expansion of the extracellular matrix,** eventually resulting in proteinuria and nephrotic syndrome. The **GBM is characteristically thickened.** Diffuse glomerulosclerosis is the most common lesion, but acellular accumulations forming the characteristic Kimmelstiel-Wilson nodules in nodular glomerulosclerosis is pathognomonic. Patients usually have a preceding diagnosis of diabetic retinopathy.

Epidemiology

African Americans, Native Americans, and Pima Indians develop nephropathy at a higher incidence than white Europeans. Males are at slightly higher risk than females. Between 15% and 20% of patients with type 2 DM and 30% and 40% of patients with type 1 DM develop nephropathy after 20 years.

Management

Aggressive glycemic control and treatment of hypertension are the mainstays of treatment. The standard of care for hypertension in patients with diabetes is **ACE inhibitors or angiotensin receptor blockers (ARBs),** which lower the rate of proteinuria and slow progression to end-stage renal disease, possibly due to both their antihypertensive effect and ability to reduce intraglomerular pressure. In early nephropathy, GFR may be increased, but with progression, GFR gradually becomes normal and continues to decrease. Nephrotic-range proteinuria occurs in 50% of patients with type 1 and type 2 diabetes. Patients with diabetes are also prone to other renal diseases, such as type IV RTA (hyporeninemic hyperaldosteronemic), papillary necrosis, and contrast material-induced nephropathy.

Complications

Diabetic nephropathy is the most common cause of end-stage renal disease in the United States, with significant associated morbidity and mortality.

Breakout Point

Diabetic "Triopathy"
• Retinopathy • Nephropathy • Neuropathy

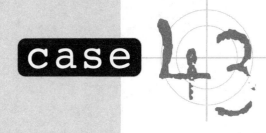

case 43

ID/CC A **25-year-old man** who presents with **blood in his urine** has been **coughing up blood** for the past several hours.

HPI He has been feeling fatigued and short of breath over the past several weeks. He has noticed blood in his urine in the past. He had URI symptoms 2 weeks ago with a chronic cough over this time, but he started coughing up blood this morning.

PE VS: **hypoxemic, tachypneic.** PE: appears fatigued; bibasilar inspiratory rales; mild edema in distal lower extremities.

Labs CBC: hypochromic, microcytic anemia **(iron deficiency anemia).** Chem 7: BUN and creatinine elevated. Urinalysis: **gross hematuria. Anti-GBM antibodies** detected in serum.

Imaging CXR: diffuse bilateral alveolar infiltrates.

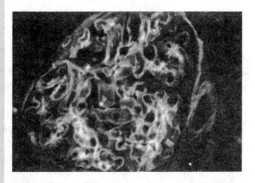

Figure 43-1. Immunofluorescence of renal biopsy: linear IgG staining on the GBM.

case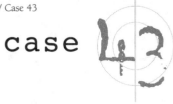

Goodpasture Syndrome

Pathogenesis

Goodpasture syndrome is an **autoimmune** disease characterized by **acute glomerulonephritis and pulmonary hemorrhage**. Pathogenesis is mediated by crossing of antibodies past the fenestrated endothelium to the glomerular (and pulmonary) basement membranes. Anti-GBM antibody binding results in inflammatory infiltration of neutrophils and macrophages, inducing a physical disruption to the glomerulus.

Epidemiology

Associated with HLA alleles. Generally rare, approximately 1 per 2 million population, and most often occurs in 20–40-year-old men.

Management

The goal of treatment is to remove the anti-GBM antibodies and also prevent resurgence of antibodies by immunosuppression. **Prednisone**, immunosuppressants, and **plasmapheresis** are recommended, and generally result in a good response. An elevated creatinine on presentation bodes a poor prognosis. Patients should be monitored for anti-GBM antibody level and creatinine trend, and they should also be salt and fluid-restricted to prevent ensuing edema.

Complications

May progress to rapidly progressive (crescentic) glomerulonephritis type I.

Breakout Point

- Hemoptysis and hematuria in young man
- Linear immunofluorescence of anti-GBM antibody binding
- Autoimmune condition; associated with HLA alleles

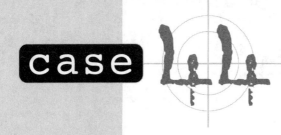

ID/CC	A **44-year-old man** with end-stage renal disease on hemodialysis complains of an **inability to move.**
HPI	The patient states that he **missed his dialysis appointment** 2 days ago. Since then he has experienced **progressive weakness.**
PE	VS: normal. PE: patient is awake, alert, and oriented ×3; lungs clear to auscultation; normal heart rate and rhythm; normal S_1 and S_2; 0/5 muscle strength in lower extremities with negative DTRs (FLACCID PARALYSIS); 1/5 strength in upper extremities; CN II–XII intact.
Labs	Lytes: **elevated potassium** (6.8 mEq/L).

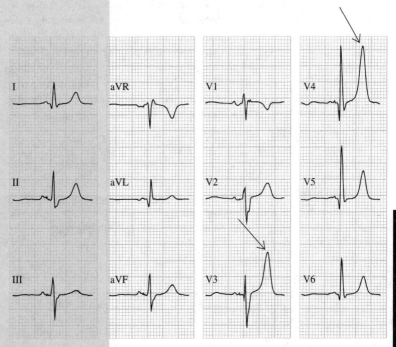

Figure 44-1. ECG: prolonged PR interval and QRS duration; peaked T waves (*arrows*).

case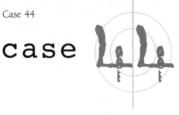

Hyperkalemia

Pathogenesis

Intracellular potassium levels are approximately 150 mEq/L, whereas extracellular levels are ordinarily about 4 mEq/L; an intracellular-to-extracellular shift may lead to profound hyperkalemia. Causes include insulin deficiency, acidosis, hyperosmolality, cell lysis, and succinylcholine therapy. Potassium levels are generally regulated by the kidney, so **derangements in renal function** (end-stage renal disease, aldosterone deficiency, aldosterone resistance) may also lead to alterations in potassium levels.

Management

ECG changes necessitate emergent **calcium gluconate** (minutes), **glucose and insulin** (20–30 minutes), **sodium bicarbonate,** and nebulized albuterol (a β2-adrenergic agonist). Stop all potassium intake. The next phase of treatment involves **potassium removal,** which may be accomplished with diuretics, dialysis, or cation exchange resins (Kayexalate). Potassium-sparing diuretics (eg, spironolactone, amiloride) should be used cautiously in patients with chronic renal failure.

Complications

Failure to treat hyperkalemia leads to progressive cardiac dysfunction, ultimately leading to VT, VF, asystole, and death.

Breakout Point

- ECG changes: peaked T waves, prolonged PR interval, wide QRS
- Immediate treatment: calcium gluconate

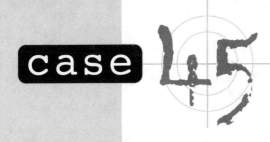

case 45

ID/CC A **52-year-old man** with rheumatoid arthritis (RA) and "borderline diabetes" presents to the outpatient clinic complaining of **abdominal bloating** and **bilateral ankle swelling** of several months' duration.

HPI The patient has suffered from severe RA for more than a decade and has been using **gold therapy** successfully for nearly 2 years. His blood sugar has been "borderline" for the past year.

PE VS: normal. PE: in no acute distress; no JVD; skin normal; lungs clear; cardiac exam normal; abdomen nontender and distended, with **positive fluid wave and shifting dullness;** extremities notable for **3+ pitting edema** in bilateral lower extremities to midcalves.

Labs CBC/Lytes: normal. UA: urine dipstick positive for 3+ protein but otherwise negative; 24-hour urine protein excretion 6.7 g/day (nephrotic range proteinuria >3.0 g/d). **Low serum albumin** (1.9 g/dL) and serum protein (5.4 g/dL); serum and urine electrophoresis negative; **hyperlipidemia.** Renal biopsy shows **thickened GBM** and **"spike and dome" pattern** with silver methenamine staining; immunofluorescence reveals finely **granular deposits of IgG and C3** along capillary loops; subepithelial electron-dense deposits seen on electron microscopy; ANA negative; TFTs normal.

case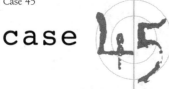

Membranous Glomerulonephritis

Pathogenesis

The precise pathogenic mechanism of membranous glomerulonephritis is unknown; it is associated with a number of disorders, including HBV, autoimmune diseases (SLE, diabetes, thyroiditis, multiple connective tissue disorders), and carcinoma, as well as with the use of drugs such as gold, penicillamine, and captopril.

Epidemiology

Membranous glomerulonephritis is the **most common cause of primary nephrotic syndrome in adults.** The male-to-female ratio is 2:1. The peak is around the fourth and fifth decades of life (almost always occurring after age 30), and an increased incidence of occult neoplasms of the lung, stomach, and colon has been observed in patients older than 50 years of age.

Management

Prednisone with or without cytotoxic agents for 3 months induces remission in some patients, but its efficacy is controversial.

Complications

Slow but progressive loss of renal function over a period of 3 to 10 years may be observed in 10% of patients. Some patients may also develop secondary renal vein thromboses as a complicating feature.

Breakout Point

- Most common nephrotic syndrome in adults
- "Spike and dome" pattern
- Associated with autoimmune disease, malignancy, and gold salts

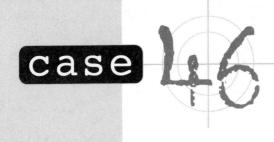

case 46

ID/CC A **7-year-old boy** presents with a 2-month history of **lower extremity edema and progressive abdominal distention.**

HPI The patient has no significant prior medical history, although he had a **"bad cold"** for several weeks that ended approximately 1 month ago. The parents deny any history of allergies, use of NSAIDs, photophobia, arthralgias, or myalgias.

PE VS: normal. PE: in no acute distress; skin normal; no JVD; thyroid normal; lungs clear; cardiopulmonary exam normal; abdomen distended, with shifting dullness and palpable fluid thrill (due to **ascites**); extremities notable for **2+ pedal** and **ankle edema** bilaterally; normal skin exam.

Labs CBC/Lytes: normal. Creatinine normal. UA: urine dipstick notable for 3+ proteinuria. **Serum albumin decreased**; serum protein decreased; **hypertriglyceridemia**; 24-hour urine protein 9.7 g/day (nephrotic-range proteinuria ≥3.0 g/day); serum and urine electrophoreses negative; ANA negative; following renal biopsy, light microscopy unremarkable; immunofluorescence negative for immunoglobulins; EM reveals **"fusion" of epithelial foot processes.**

Imaging US, abdomen: excess peritoneal fluid (ASCITES).

case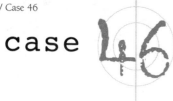

Minimal-Change Disease

Pathogenesis

The precise etiology of minimal-change disease remains unknown. It is associated with **recent viral URIs,** immunizations, hypersensitivity reactions to drugs (eg, NSAIDs), or allergic reactions (eg, bee stings), and it may also occur as a paraneoplastic manifestation of Hodgkin disease.

Epidemiology

Minimal-change disease is the **most common cause of nephrotic syndrome in children** but is occasionally seen in adults.

Management

Prednisone induces remission in 50% of adults and in 90% of children, but more than 50% of patients relapse. Add cyclophosphamide or chlorambucil for relapsed disease. Diuretics are used to decrease severe edema. Although patients with minimal-change disease rarely progress to renal failure, they often develop complications requiring monitoring.

Complications

Increased susceptibility to bacterial infections (gram-positive organisms), spontaneous bacterial peritonitis, thromboembolic events, severe hyperlipidemia, and protein malnutrition.

Breakout Point

- Most common cause of nephrotic syndrome in children
- Responsive to corticosteroids (prednisone)
- Normal glomerulus on light microscopy
- Fusion of epithelial foot processes on electron microscopy

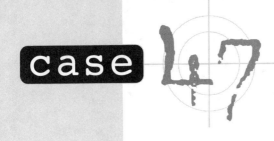

case 47

ID/CC   A **35-year-old man** presents with severe flank pain that he has had **for the past hour.**

HPI   He was awakened this morning by **sudden** severe right flank pain that **radiates toward his right groin;** the pain comes in **episodic attacks.** He **vomited** twice and had dark urine this morning. He states that he has not been drinking fluids much because he has been busy at work.

PE   VS: hypertensive, tachycardic, tachypneic. PE: **writhing around the bed in pain;** severe costovertebral tenderness is elicited with palpation; abdomen is soft with no suprapubic tenderness; testes normally descended bilaterally.

Labs   UA: positive for RBC and calcium, with high specific gravity. CBC: normal. Serum uric acid, calcium, PTH normal.

Imaging   KUB: **radiopaque density at ureteropelvic junction.**

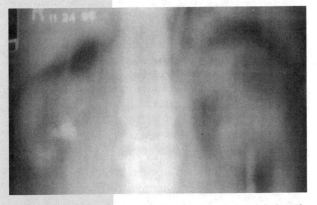

Figure 47-1. KUB: **radiopaque density at ureteropelvic junction.**

case 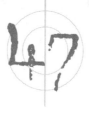 47

Nephrolithiasis

Pathogenesis

There are five types of urinary calculi: **calcium oxalate, calcium phosphate, struvite, cystine, and uric acid.** Calculi are polycrystalline aggregates that form due to conditions dependent on pH, solute concentration, and nidus formation. **Dehydration,** high sodium dietary intake, and living in hot temperate regions are predisposing factors. Rare genetic disorders such as cystinuria can predispose to cystine stones. The most common stones are composed of calcium; thus 85% of stones are radiopaque. Uric acid stones are radiolucent (which may not show up on KUB and may require CT abdomen for identification) and may occur in patients with gout or hyperuricemia.

Epidemiology

Extremely common, approximately 300,000–700,000 per year. The male-to-female ratio is 3:1. They occur most commonly in the third to fourth decades.

Management

Standard of care is **IV fluids and NSAIDs such as ketorolac** (which decrease inflammation and have a ureteral relaxing effect). **Twenty-four–hour urine collection for levels of pH, calcium, oxalate, uric acid, sodium, phosphorus, citrate, magnesium, creatinine, and total volume should be obtained,** because treatment is determined by type of stone. Urinary calculi containing calcium cannot be dissolved with current therapy and are usually spontaneously passed in the urine, treated with **extracorporeal shock wave lithotripsy,** or physically extracted in percutaneous nephrostomy. Calculi containing uric acid can be dissolved by alkalinization of the urine with sodium bicarbonate or potassium citrate administration. Consistent intake of fluids, limiting sodium intake to 100 mEq/d, and bran (decreases urinary calcium by binding calcium and decreasing bowel transit time) should be encouraged. Decreasing calcium intake is not recommended.

Complications

Prognosis is generally good, but in severe cases, obstruction can lead to pyelonephritis and urosepsis.

Breakout Point

- Sudden-onset colicky flank pain and hematuria
- Writhing in pain (versus peritonitis)

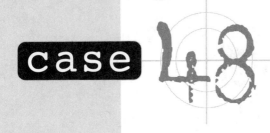

case 48

ID/CC	A 25-year-old man presents with blood in his urine.
HPI	He had one episode of painless **dark brown ("cola-colored") urine** and puffiness around his eyes that started this morning. He reports URI symptoms and sore throat 2 weeks ago but has since recovered fully.
PE	VS: **hypertensive.** PE: well-appearing; periorbital edema; diffuse mild pitting edema; lungs clear.
Labs	UA: **tea-colored, RBC positive, red cell casts, protein 2.5 g/d.** CBC: normal. Chem 7: elevated BUN and creatinine. Streptozyme test positive (**antistreptolysin O, anti-DNase B,** antihyaluronidase, antinicotinamide adenine dinucleotidase titers). **C3 and C4 low** (indicates presence of antigen–antibody complexes).
Imaging	US, kidneys: normal. **Light microscopy: hypercellularity of glomeruli** with PMN and monocyte infiltration. **Immunofluorescence: "lumpy-bumpy" granular deposits of IgG and C3.** EM: electron-dense "humps" (immune complex deposits) on the epithelial side (subepithelial location) of the basement membrane.

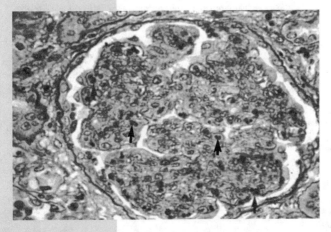

Figure 48-1. Light microscopy: hypercellularity of glomeruli with PMN and monocyte infiltration (*arrows*).

case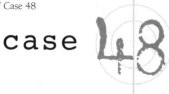

Postinfectious Glomerulonephritis

Pathogenesis

Postinfectious glomerulonephritis, also called post-streptococcal glomerulonephritis, can **occur 1 to 3 weeks after nephritogenic strains causing Group A β-hemolytic streptococcus (GABHS) pharyngitis, impetigo,** tonsillitis, or insect bites. The etiology is unclear but may be deposition of streptococcal antigens in the basement membrane, which precipitates subepithelial antibody–antigen complex formation.

Epidemiology

Can occur sporadically or in epidemics, especially in developing countries. More common in males, primarily at 2–15 years of age, but may occur in adults.

Management

Supportive care, including antihypertensives and diuretics. Antibiotics are generally ineffective unless streptococcal pharyngitis or impetigo is ongoing. Corticosteroids do not improve outcome. Considered benign in children but may induce severe azotemia, CHF, and crescent formation in adults.

Complications

Five percent of adults develop rapidly progressive glomerulonephritis and chronic renal insufficiency.

Breakout Point

- Tea-colored urine with red cell casts
- Hypercellularity of glomeruli on light microscopy
- "Lumpy-bumpy" immunofluorescence
- "Humps" on electron microscopy
- Occurs 1–3 weeks after pharyngitis or impetigo

case 49

ID/CC   A **73-year-old man** with adult-onset **DM,** hypertension, and RA presents with a decline in **mental status** and **decreased urinary output.**

HPI   The patient has been diabetic for nearly 30 years, with poorly controlled blood sugar despite insulin and oral agents; he has had **ocular disease** and **renal insufficiency** for more than 5 years. He currently takes ACE inhibitors, a thiazide diuretic, and calcium channel blockers for hypertension and takes **NSAIDs** for persistent RA. He denies any asthma.

PE   VS: no fever (37.1°C); tachycardia (HR 119); tachypnea (RR 28); hypertension (BP 140/84). PE: disoriented; lethargic, moderately responsive, and in mild distress.

Labs   CBC: normal. Lytes: **hyperkalemia; hyperchloremia. Elevated BUN and creatinine.** ABGs: **non–anion gap metabolic acidosis.** UA: acidic urine (pH <5.5); **urinary anion gap positive;** proximal H^+ secretion normal.

Imaging   None.

case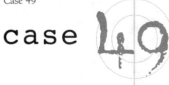

Renal Tubular Acidosis

Pathogenesis

RTA results from deficient H^+ secretion in the distal tubule (**type I**), defective bicarbonate reabsorption in the proximal tubule (**type II**), and defective secretion of both potassium and H^+ in the distal nephron (**type IV**). Type IV is due to a generalized distal nephron dysfunction attributable to either insufficient aldosterone production or intrinsic renal disease, causing **aldosterone resistance**; the resulting hyperkalemia decreases proximal tubule ammonia production and reduces H^+ secretion, leading to inadequate excretion of the acid load. These patients produce acidic urine despite reduced H^+ secretion because of inadequate ammonia to buffer the protons in the distal tubule. RTA is diagnosed by laboratory evidence of primary metabolic acidosis, a normal serum anion gap (<12), a zero or positive urine anion gap, and exclusion of the presence of diarrhea, calcium chloride, or other acids.

Epidemiology

Whereas types I and II RTA are rare, **type IV RTA is a common cause of normal anion gap metabolic acidosis.** It is seen most commonly in patients with **renal insufficiency** and chronic medical illnesses such as **DM** (with nephropathy), **tubular interstitial renal disease, hypertension,** and AIDS. Drugs such as **NSAIDs, ACE inhibitors, and heparin** can also produce or contribute to type IV RTA.

Management

Restrict dietary potassium; discontinue aldosterone antagonists (NSAIDs, ACE inhibitors, heparin). Mineralocorticoid replacement with **fludrocortisone** usually improves hyperkalemia and acidosis but may worsen hypertension; patients with tubular resistance require higher doses, whereas hypertension and CHF are relative contraindications. **Loop diuretics**, sodium bicarbonate, and exchange resins can also be used. Acidosis generally improves as the hyperkalemic contribution to decreased ammonia production is corrected.

Complications

Complications of type IV RTA are those of metabolic acidosis and hyperkalemia, including confusion, weakness, paresthesias, paralysis, arrhythmias, and even cardiac arrest when severe.

Breakout Point

- Types I and II RTA are rare
- Type IV RTA is a common cause of normal anion gap metabolic acidosis, resulting from aldosterone deficiency or resistance
- Type IV RTA is prevalent in patients with DM, interstitial renal disease, hypertension, and AIDS

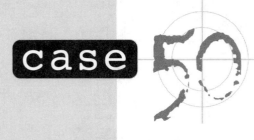

case 50

ID/CC	A **28-year-old white woman** presents to the clinic for a routine physical exam.
HPI	On questioning, she notes that she has been urinating more frequently than normal and does not feel as strong as she once did (**polyuria** and **muscle weakness** secondary to hypokalemia caused by hyperaldosteronism).
PE	VS: hypertension (BP 190/100). PE: thin and well developed; **loud, high-pitched, epigastric bruit bilaterally.**
Labs	ABGs: **metabolic alkalosis.** Lytes: hypokalemia (3.0 mEq/L). Captopril test reveals exaggerated plasma renin activity.
Imaging	US, renal artery (duplex): bilateral renal artery stenosis >50%.

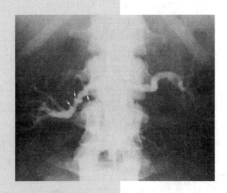

Figure 50-1. Angio, renal: **"string of beads"** (alternating thick fibromuscular ridges and thin vessel wall) appearance of the right renal artery (*arrows*) (a different case).

case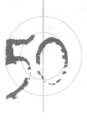

Renovascular Hypertension: Fibromuscular Dysplasia

Pathogenesis

Fibromuscular dysplasia is a **disease of small and medium-sized arteries** that is characterized most commonly by **medial hyperplasia with or without elastic membrane fibrosis** (MEDIAL DYSPLASIA). Periadventitial or intimal dysplasia may also be observed. Resulting renal artery stenosis causes decreased perfusion to the kidney, with subsequent activation of the renin–angiotensin–aldosterone axis. This hormonal activation results in hypertension (action of angiotensin II and volume expansion due to aldosterone) and electrolyte abnormalities secondary to hyperaldosteronism (hypernatremia, hypokalemia, and metabolic alkalosis). Polyuria may result from severe hypokalemia. The right renal artery is involved more frequently than the left.

Epidemiology

This disorder most commonly arises in **females** and **frequently affects the renal and carotid arteries.** It may, however, involve peripheral vasculature, producing symptoms similar to peripheral vascular disease. It is rare in blacks.

Management

Percutaneous transluminal angioplasty (cures more than 50% of patients); medical management of hypertension (ACE inhibitors).

Complications

Renal scarring secondary to ischemia.

Breakout Point

- Presents as hypertension in a young female
- "String of beads" appearance to renal artery

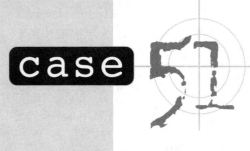

case

ID/CC	A **29-year-old woman** complains of **pain on urination** (DYSURIA).
HPI	Directed questioning reveals that the patient has also experienced increased urinary **frequency** and **urgency.**
PE	VS: normal. PE: mild suprapubic tenderness; no costovertebral angle tenderness.
Labs	UA: **leukocyte esterase and nitrate positive; pyuria** without WBC casts; urine culture reveals >10^5 CFU/mL; gram-negative bacilli identified as *Escherichia coli*.
Imaging	None.

case 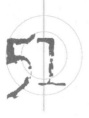 51

Urinary Tract Infection

Pathogenesis

Most UTIs result from bacteria ascending into the bladder from the urethra. **E. coli** is responsible for most (80%) cases of acute infections in patients without catheters, calculi, or urologic abnormalities. Other gram-negative rods, including **Proteus**, **Klebsiella**, and **Enterobacter**, are responsible for a smaller number of infections. Gram-positive cocci (eg, **Staphylococcus saprophyticus**) also play a role in producing UTIs in sexually active women. UTIs are generally categorized as catheter-associated (usually nosocomial) or non–catheter-associated infections. UTIs may also be classified as those affecting the lower urinary tract (cystitis, urethritis, prostatitis) and those affecting the upper tract (pyelonephritis). Alkaline urine suggests the presence of a urea-splitting organism (most commonly **Proteus**).

Epidemiology

The incidence of UTIs increases with the onset of sexual activity. They are more **prevalent during pregnancy** because of the decreased ureteral tone/ureteral peristalsis and temporary incompetence of the vesicoureteral valves. 10–20% of the elderly population and up to 50% of institutionalized elderly persons have bacteriuria.

Management

TMP-SMX is considered the **first-line** regimen in areas where resistance of E. coli is low. **Predisposing factors** such as **vesicoureteral reflux, obstruction, neurogenic bladder,** or **calculi** should be identified and treated if possible. Recurrent infections should be identified to determine whether the same strain or a different strain is responsible for recurrence; patients with repeated infections or recent hospitalizations may harbor resistant strains. Individuals with recurrent infection (more than three infections per year) benefit from daily long-term administration of TMP-SMX. Recommend that patients urinate following sexual intercourse.

Complications

Treatment commonly results in complete resolution of symptoms. Permanent renal damage may result with ascending infection and resultant pyelonephritis.

Breakout Point

- Treat asymptomatic bacteriuria only in pregnant women and with GU tract instrumentation
- Second most common cause in young healthy women is *Staphylococcus saprophyticus*

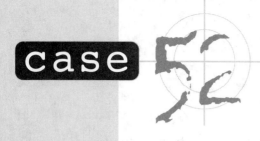

ID/CC A 47-year-old man complains of **severe shortness of breath.**

HPI The patient was admitted 2 days ago for acute pancreatitis.

PE VS: **fever** (38.5°C); **tachycardia** (HR 112); **tachypnea** (RR 30–36); hypotension. PE: altered mental status; **central cyanosis;** warm, moist skin; accessory muscles (sternocleidomastoid and scalenes) used for respiration with intercostal retractions (respiratory distress); **bilateral inspiratory rales** and coarse breath sounds.

Labs CBC: leukocytosis. ABGs: **severe hypoxemia** (<70 mm Hg) **refractory to increased FIo_2; Pao_2-to-FIo_2 ratio less than 200:1.** Swan–Ganz catheter reveals **pulmonary capillary wedge pressure <18 mm Hg** (noncardiogenic pulmonary edema); elevated amylase and lipase.

Imaging CXR: **diffuse bilateral alveolar and interstitial infiltrates** with normal heart size. Echo: **normal LV function.**

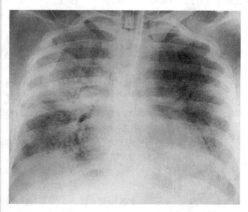

Figure 52-1. CXR: Diffuse bilateral fluffy infiltrates.

103

case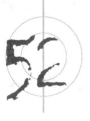

Adult Respiratory Distress Syndrome

Pathogenesis

ARDS represents a common pathway for many pathologic processes (sepsis, shock, massive trauma, DIC, pneumonia, burns, oxygen toxicity, emboli) that lead to **increased capillary permeability** and consequent **extravasation of intraluminal contents into the interstitium and eventually the alveoli,** leading to pulmonary edema and atelectasis. The presence of vascular contents, especially fibrinogen, within the alveoli leads to **deranged surfactant production and fibrinolysis,** allowing for the formation of **hyaline membranes.** Eventually, this leads to **decreased lung compliance,** requiring greater inspiratory pressures, which translates into increased work of breathing.

Management

Endotracheal intubation and **mechanical ventilation** with PEEP and **supplemental oxygen; IV fluids** for hypotension; DVT prophylaxis (SC heparin). **Nutritional supplementation** is needed because patients have an increased basal metabolism. **Antibiotics** for treatment of underlying sepsis.

Complications

Patients often suffer from multisystem organ failure, DIC, sepsis, or shock. ARDS ultimately leads to death in **50% to 60% of cases.** Patients who do survive generally recover 90% of their previous pulmonary function within the first year, but they may suffer oxygen toxicity secondary to long-term administration of $>50\%$ FIO_2. Complications of PEEP include spontaneous pneumothorax and reduced cardiac output.

Breakout Point

- Acute onset of respiratory failure after traumatic event
- Bilateral white fluffy infiltrates on CXR
- Absence of elevated left atrial pressure
- PaO_2-to-FIO_2 <200, regardless of PEEP

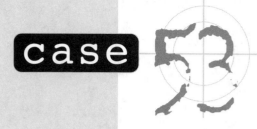

ID/CC A 69-year-old white man who is a retired **shipyard worker** complains of a feeling of **breathlessness, initially on exertion and now even at rest.**

HPI The patient states that he worked for over **30 years in construction,** focusing primarily on the restoration of **old buildings.** He states that he has had a dry cough for years along with worsening fatigue, anorexia, and weight loss. He denies any history of smoking.

PE VS: no fever; tachycardia (HR 115); tachypnea (RR 30); normal BP. PE: clubbing; **dry end inspiratory fine bibasilar crackles;** loud P_2, parasternal heave (RVH) and JVD (secondary to pulmonary hypertension).

Labs Sputum examination reveals **asbestos bodies.** PFTs: **reduced total lung capacity, vital capacity, residual volume, and DL_{CO};** normal FEV_1/FVC.

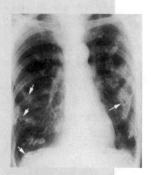

Figure 53-1. CXR: ground-glass appearance and small linear opacities (septal lines) most pronounced at bases.

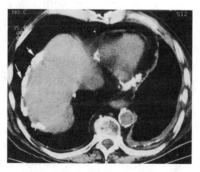

Figure 53-2. CT, chest: demonstrates calcified pleural plaques, especially over the right hemidiaphragm.

case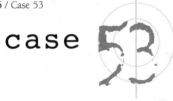

Asbestosis

Pathogenesis

Asbestosis is a **diffuse interstitial fibrosing disease** that follows prolonged inhalation of any asbestiform fiber. Alveolar macrophages phagocytose these fibers and undergo membrane damage. Lysosomal enzymes are subsequently liberated, damaging the parenchyma of the lung, which heals by **scarring** and **fibrosis** and produces diffuse interstitial fibrosis. With advanced disease, the acinar units are eventually obliterated, forming a "**honeycombed lung.**" Asbestos-related pleural disease is the most common manifestation of chronic exposure to asbestos and is completely benign.

Epidemiology

Asbestosis occurs primarily in individuals who have at least 10 years of moderate to severe **exposure to asbestos,** usually in the workplace (miners, shipyard workers, boilermakers, mill workers), and there is a 20- to 30-year **latency period.** Asbestos exposure is also associated with an increased risk of **malignant mesothelioma** (both pleural and peritoneal) and **lung cancer** (increased risk in chronic smokers).

Management

There is no definitive treatment for asbestosis or mesothelioma; thus, pulmonary physiotherapy, **elimination of exposure**, and **smoking cessation** are crucial.

Complications

Among patients with a history of cigarette smoking, the incidence of both **SCC** and **adenocarcinoma of the lung** is elevated approximately **55-fold.** Death usually occurs with onset of asbestosis-related symptoms within 12 to 24 months and may be earlier if Caplan syndrome, pulmonary hypertension, or cor pulmonale develops.

Breakout Point

- Prevalent in shipyard workers and miners
- Asbestos rods are described as ferruginous bodies
- Predisposes to malignant mesothelioma

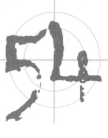

case 54

ID/CC A **30-year-old man** presents to the ED with an acute attack of **shortness of breath, coughing,** and **wheezing.**

HPI He has a history of asthma from childhood. He states the attack occurred several hours after playing with a neighbor's cat.

PE VS: no fever; **tachycardia** (HR 130); **tachypnea** (RR 40); PE: **confused** and **diaphoretic; uses accessory muscles** of respiration; cyanosis; lungs hyperresonant to percussion; inspiratory and expiratory **diffuse wheezing** bilaterally; increased E-to-I ratio.

Labs CBC: **eosinophilia.** ABGs: primary **respiratory alkalosis** with **reduced P_{O_2} and P_{CO_2}** (elevated P_{CO_2} indicates respiratory failure); **peak flows decreased.** PFTs: **low FEV_1/FVC** with >15% improvement of FEV_1 following administration of β_2-agonist; sputum analysis reveals **Curschmann spirals** (mucus that forms casts in small airways) and **Charcot–Leyden crystals** (eosinophil breakdown products); elevated serum IgE.

Imaging CXR: hyperinflation, flattened diaphragms (secondary to air trapping and increased residual volume).

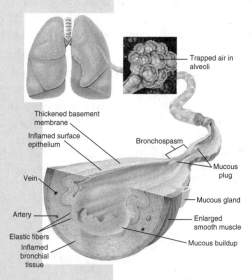

Figure 54-1. Pathogenesis of asthma.

case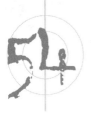

Asthma: Chronic

Pathogenesis

Bronchial asthma is characterized by airway constriction secondary to reversible, episodic contractions of airway smooth muscle due to **hyperreactivity**, hypersecretion of **tenacious mucus,** and **mucosal edema** (due to inflammation). It may occur as a response to an allergen **(type I hypersensitivity reaction)** or may be **intrinsic.** Acute attacks may be precipitated by cold air or pollution, allergens, smoking, airway infections, emotional stress, and exercise.

Epidemiology

Afflicts 4% to 5% of the population. Children often have the **atopic** form (which may remit in the second decade), whereas intrinsic and occupational asthma arises more commonly in adults.

Management

Manage acute exacerbations with O_2, appropriate respiratory support (including mechanical ventilation if necessary), nebulized β_2-agonists (eg, albuterol) and ipratropium, systemic steroids, and antibiotics if indicated in cases with underlying infection. Prophylactic therapy may include **inhaled corticosteroids** (beclomethasone), cromolyn sodium (particularly in children with extrinsic asthma), **leukotriene inhibitors,** and, in severe cases, oral steroids.

Complications

Asthma may lead to **unremitting bronchospasm** (status asthmaticus), **respiratory failure,** respiratory arrest, and death. Patients are also prone to develop recurrent respiratory infections and pneumothorax.

Breakout Point

- Symptoms worse at night or early in morning
- Prolonged expiratory wheeze
- Positive bronchoprovocation test
- Curschmann spirals and Charcot-Leyden crystals in lungs

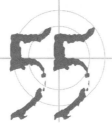

case 55

ID/CC	A 56-year-old man presents with shortness of breath and a chronic cough productive of copious mucoid sputum.
HPI	Over the past 3 years, his symptoms have occurred for at least 3 months of every year. He also reports a 40-pack-year smoking history.
PE	VS: tachypnea (RR 25). PE: blue lips (CENTRAL CYANOSIS); plethora; bilateral rhonchi and wheezes.
Labs	CBC: hematocrit increased. ABGs: hypoxia and hypercapnia. ECG: presence of P pulmonale and poor progression of R wave in chest leads. PFTs: obstructive pattern of increased residual volume and decreased FEV_1/FVC.
Imaging	CXR, PA: presence of increased basilar bronchovascular markings and thickened bronchial walls.

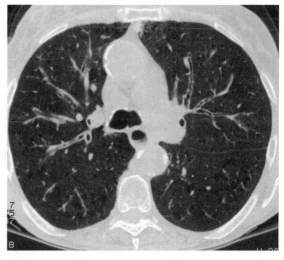

Figure 55-1. CT, chest: mild bronchial dilation and mural thickening.

case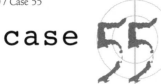

Chronic Obstructive Pulmonary Disease: Chronic Bronchitis

Pathogenesis

The pathologic hallmark of chronic bronchitis is **enlargement of the mucous glands** in the major bronchi. The diameter of the mucous glands relative to the thickness of the bronchial wall (the Reid index) is typically increased from values of 0.26 to 0.44 in healthy persons to more than 0.50 in patients with chronic bronchitis. **Smoking** and **occupational exposure** to harmful substances are the principal etiologic factors.

Epidemiology

Seen primarily in smokers.

Management

Smoking cessation and long-term administration of **supplemental oxygen** are the two most important interventions. **Bronchodilators, antibiotics, and corticosteroids** may be used in acute exacerbations.

Complications

Cor pulmonale.

Breakout Point

- "Blue bloater"
- History of cigarette smoking
- Chronic cough for 3 months or more in at least two consecutive years
- Chronic sputum production

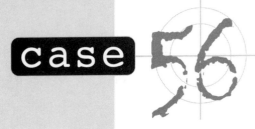

ID/CC   A **60-year-old man** complains of progressive **shortness of breath on exertion** and a **nonproductive cough.**

HPI   He has a 60-pack-year **smoking history.**

PE   VS: no fever; **tachypnea** (RR 24). PE: moderate **respiratory distress; pursed lips;** using **accessory muscles** of respiration; **barrel-shaped chest; hyperresonant percussion** note; distant breath sounds; scattered rhonchi heard bilaterally on auscultation; heart sounds distant.

Labs   ABGs: mild hypoxia with hypocapnia. PFTs: **decreased FEV$_1$/FVC ratio;** decreased DL$_{CO}$; increased TLC, FRC, and RV.

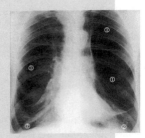

Figure 56-1. CXR, PA: hypertranslucent lung fields with large bullae (1); flattening of the diaphragm (2), and elongated tubular heart shadow.

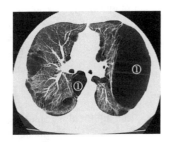

Figure 56-2. CT, chest: multiple large bullae (1).

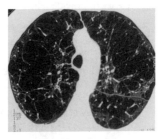

Figure 56-3. CT, chest: innumerable smaller bullae.

111

case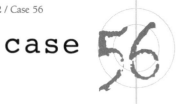

Chronic Obstructive Pulmonary Disease: Emphysema

Pathogenesis

Emphysema is abnormal permanent **enlargement of air spaces distal to the terminal bronchiole** accompanied by the **destruction of the alveolar walls.** It may involve the acinus and the lobule uniformly (panacinar) or may primarily involve the respiratory bronchioles (centriacinar). **Panacinar** emphysema is common in patients with α_1-**antitrypsin** deficiency. Typically, the lower lobes show more involvement than the upper lobes. **Centriacinar** emphysema is commonly found in **cigarette smokers** and is rare in nonsmokers. It is usually more extensive and severe in the upper lobes. Emphysema leads to a **reduction in elastic recoil** in the lung that leads to narrowing of the airways with a subsequent decrease in expiratory flow rates (airway obstruction).

Epidemiology

CAO is a leading cause of death in the United States and is second only to CAD as a Social Security–compensated disability. Between **80% and 90% of cases of CAO can be attributed to cigarette smoking;** a small percentage is attributable to α_1-**antitrypsin deficiency.** The risk of death from emphysema or chronic bronchitis is 30 times greater for heavy smokers (>25 cigarettes/day) than for nonsmokers.

Management

Smoking cessation and long-term administration of **supplemental oxygen** are the two most important interventions. **Bronchodilators** are commonly used; **antibiotics** in acute exacerbations; **corticosteroids** in resistant cases. Influenza and pneumococcal vaccines are recommended. Lung volume reduction surgery and lung transplantation are promising treatments. Surgical excision of bullae may be necessary to provide relief.

Complications

Chronic hypoxemia causes **secondary erythrocytosis** and contributes to exercise limitation, pulmonary hypertension, right heart failure, spontaneous pneumothorax from rupturing of blebs and bullae, and impaired neuropsychiatric function.

Breakout Point

- "Pink puffer"
- History of cigarette smoking
- Decreased FEV_1/FVC ratio

case 57

ID/CC An **18-year-old man** presents with refractory **myopia** and **scoliosis**.

HPI He complains that his schoolmates make fun of his **exceptionally long arms, fingers, and legs**.

PE VS: normal. PE: slit-lamp exam shows **ectopia lentis** (lens dislocation); moderate **chest wall depression** (PECTUS EXCAVATUM); marked **scoliosis**; midsystolic click and soft 2/6 systolic murmur (mitral valve prolapse) audible at apex with radiation to axilla; aortic diastolic murmur (aortic insufficiency), limbs long and thin with **increased arm span**; moderate **arachnodactyly**.

Labs Normal.

Imaging Echo: **mitral valve prolapse** with mild mitral valve insufficiency and mild **aortic root dilatation** with mild aortic insufficiency.

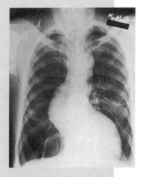

Figure 57-1. CXR: Aortic dissection affecting the ascending aorta.

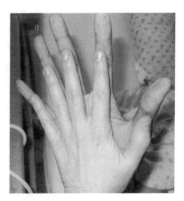

Figure 57-2. Arach no dactyly, & hands/fingers are elongated and spidery.

case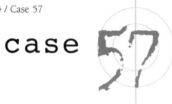

Marfan Syndrome

Pathogenesis

Marfan syndrome is an **autosomal dominant** connective tissue disease that results from **a mutation in the fibrillin gene** (chromosome 15). Fibrillin is a 350-kDa glycoprotein that serves as a major component of elastin-associated microfibrils abundant in large blood vessels and the suspensory ligaments of the lens. **Cystic medial necrosis** of the aorta (predisposing to dissection) and **myxomatous cardiac valve** (usually aortic and mitral) disease are classical abnormalities.

Epidemiology

Marfan syndrome occurs in 1 in 10,000 persons. Approximately 25% of patients have no affected parents; these are usually due to a new mutation. It affects both genders equally.

Management

Regular ophthalmologic surveillance (follow closely for visual acuity to prevent amblyopia and retinal detachment); **annual orthopedic consultation** to ensure early diagnosis of scoliosis; annual echocardiography to monitor aortic diameter and mitral valve function; **endocarditis prophylaxis.** Beta-adrenergic blockade to retard the rate of aortic dilatation; restrict significant physical activity to protect against aortic dissection. **Prophylactic replacement of the aortic root** with composite graft should be considered when the diameter approaches 50 to 55 mm (normal <40 mm).

Complications

Mitral valve prolapse typically develops early in life and can result in mitral insufficiency (the most common cause of death in children); aortic root dilatation can result in aortic regurgitation, aortic dissection, or aortic rupture. **Ectopia lentis** is a central diagnostic feature that results in cataract formation, ocular globe elongation, and retinal detachment. **Spontaneous pneumothoraces** secondary to multiple thoracic cage deformities (pectus excavatum, scoliosis) as well as **inguinal and incisional hernias** are common. In untreated patients, mortality may result in the fourth or fifth decade due to aortic dissection or **CHF** secondary to aortic regurgitation.

Breakout Point

- Autosomal dominant
- Mutations in the fibrillin-1 (FBN-1) gene
- Aortic dilation, aortic dissection, and mitral valve prolapse
- Arm span/height ratio is >1.05 (arms/legs disproportionately longer than torso)
- Associated with pectus excavatum, scoliosis, ectopia lentis (lens dislocation), and arachnodactyly

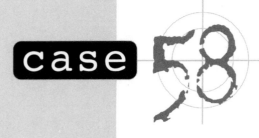

ID/CC An **obese 40-year-old man** presents with daytime sleepiness.

HPI His wife states that he **snores loudly** at night, has episodes in which he **stops breathing for a full 30 seconds while sleeping and suddenly wakes up with a loud snort and gasping, and sleeps very restlessly** and thrashes around in bed. He often falls asleep sitting up in the middle of conversations, and he states that he is chronically **fatigued**.

PE VS: **oxygen saturation 89% on room air.** PE: obese, falls asleep during history-taking but is easily arousable; oropharynx is narrowed with **excessive soft tissue skin folds and large uvula; neck circumference is 17.5 in;** lungs clear bilaterally.

Labs CBC: erythrocytosis. Serum and urine toxin screen negative. ABG: mildly decreased pH, hypoxia, hypercapnia.

Imaging None.

```
                        Sleep Apnea
                   Wake        Sleep        Wake
Type               ├────────┼──────────┼────────┤
Obstructive apnea
    Airflow
    Respiratory effort
Mixed apnea
    Airflow
    Respiratory effort
Central apnea
    Airflow
    Respiratory effort
Hypopnea
    Airflow
    Respiratory effort
```

Figure 58-1. Polysomnography demonstrating mixed apnea, central apnea, and hypopnea.

115

case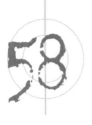

Obstructive Sleep Apnea

Pathogenesis

Obstructive sleep apnea is characterized by recurrent episodes of airway obstruction during sleep. Loss of normal pharyngeal muscle tone leads to **pharyngeal collapse** during inspiration; obstruction is exacerbated by excessive pharyngeal soft tissue. Obesity, anatomically narrowed airways, alcohol or sedative intake before sleep, hypothyroidism, cigarette smoking, and male gender are predisposing factors.

Epidemiology

This is a common condition in the United States, affecting 10%–20% of men and 5%–10% of women.

Management

Polysomnography may reveal apneic episodes that last 30–60 seconds and may demonstrate marked hypoxemia and bradydysrhythmias. **Weight loss** (10%–20% of body weight), avoidance of alcohol or sedative intake, and sleeping on the side are the first steps in management, but these goals usually cannot be achieved or are insufficient alone. The standard of care is **nasal CPAP**, which is very effective for most patients, but has a low compliance due to discomfort. **Uvulopalatopharyngoplasty** is surgical or laser resection of excess pharyngeal soft tissue and is effective in 50% of appropriate patients.

Complications

Severe obstructive sleep apnea is a significant risk factor for hypertension, nonfatal myocardial infarct, and CVA. Associated disorders, such as obesity hypoventilation syndrome or metabolic syndrome, can lead to pulmonary hypertension or cardiovascular morbidity.

Breakout Point

- Daytime somnolence
- Loud snoring with apneic events
- Polysomnography shows apnea with hypoxemia

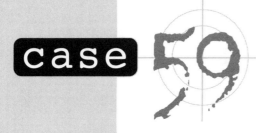

ID/CC A **65-year-old man** with a history of CHF presents with dyspnea, chest pain, **and** leg swelling **for the past 2 weeks.**

HPI He reports a **nonproductive cough** and dyspnea with little exertion. Chest pain is **sharp, stabbing, and worse with inspiration or cough.** His leg swelling has been getting progressively worse. He was traveling out of town for the past 2 weeks and forgot to take his daily diuretic medication during that time.

PE VS: **tachypnea, tachycardia, hypoxemia.** PE: increased work of breathing; diffuse rales bilaterally; **dullness to percussion, decreased breath sounds bilaterally in lung bases, decreased tactile fremitus, E to A change (egophony);** S_3 and S_4 present; moderate pitting edema in lower extremities.

Labs CBC/Lytes: mild hyponatremia.

Imaging CXR: bilateral pleural effusions. Thoracentesis: pleural fluid sample shows pH 7.40, few WBCs, few RBCs, glucose equal to serum glucose, low LDH, low protein.

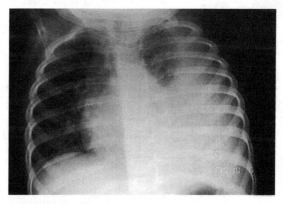

Figure 59-1. CXR: bilateral pleural effusions.

117

case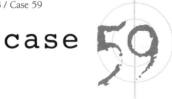

Pleural Effusion

Pathogenesis

Pleural effusion is defined as an abnormal collection of fluid in the pleural space. Fluid type may include serous **transudate (low protein)** (CHF, cirrhosis, renal failure), **exudate (high protein)** (empyema, malignancy), blood (hemothorax), and lipid/lymph (chylothorax). Transudative pleural effusions occur in the setting of increased hydrostatic pressure (CHF) or decreased oncotic pressure (hypoalbuminemia, cirrhosis).

Epidemiology

Pleural effusion affects over 1 million patients per year. **The most common causes of pleural effusion are CHF (by far), pneumonia, hypoalbuminemia, pulmonary embolus, pancreatitis, and malignancy.**

Management

The type of pleural effusion is determined first by collecting a pleural fluid sample via **thoracentesis.** Pleural fluid is analyzed for pH, CBC with differential, glucose, LDH, and protein. To distinguish between an exudate and transudate, the following criteria are used. An exudate is defined as **(1) ratio of pleural fluid protein to serum protein >0.5, (2) ratio of pleural fluid LDH to serum LDH >0.6, and (3) pleural fluid LDH greater than the upper limit of normal serum LDH.** This case presents a transudative effusion due to decompensated CHF. In pleural effusion, the treatment is determined by the underlying etiology.

Complications

Infection, multilobar involvement, and respiratory insufficiency.

Breakout Point

- Classically presents as dyspnea and pleuritic chest pain
- Dullness to percussion, decreased breath sounds, egophony
- Distinguish transudate versus exudate for underlying etiology

case 60

ID/CC A **38-year-old man** presents to the outpatient clinic with complaints of **acute-onset** right-sided **chest pain** and **shortness of breath** that started yesterday afternoon.

HPI The pain and dyspnea are localized to the right side, are unrelated to position or activity, and actually started while the patient was resting. His symptoms have been stable over the past day, and he has had no progressive difficulty breathing. He has no prior medical or family history but reports that he has **smoked** approximately one pack of cigarettes per day for 10 years.

PE VS: mild tachycardia. PE: **tall and thin**; in mild distress; no JVD or lymphadenopathy; **diminished breath sounds, decreased tactile fremitus,** and **hyperresonance** in right lung fields; no mediastinal or tracheal shift or cyanosis noted; cardiac exam normal.

Labs ABGs: **hypoxemia,** acute respiratory alkalosis. ECG: unremarkable.

Imaging See Figures 60-1 and 60-2.

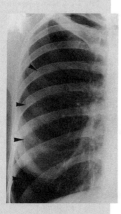

Figure 60-1. CXR: the diagnostic **visceral pleural line** is seen on the right side (*arrow*) peripheral to this, the area is seen to be **hyperlucent,** because the lung has retracted.

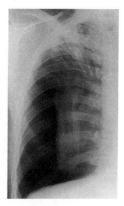

Figure 60-2. CXR: Hyperlvcent area surrounding the viseeral plevval line.

119

case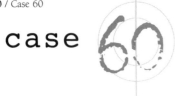

Pneumothorax: Spontaneous

Pathogenesis

Pneumothorax represents an accumulation of air in the pleural space and is classified as spontaneous or traumatic. It is believed to occur as a result of the **rupture of subpleural apical blebs** in response to **high negative intrapleural pressure.** Spontaneous pneumothorax is most commonly primary (without an underlying cause) but may be secondary to pre-existing pulmonary disease (COPD, asthma, CF, TB) and occurs predominantly in smokers. Traumatic pneumothorax results from penetrating or nonpenetrating trauma, often from iatrogenic causes (eg, thoracocentesis, pleural biopsy, positive-pressure mechanical ventilation).

Epidemiology

Pneumothorax typically affects **tall, thin men** in their **third and fourth decades.** Prior history of *Pneumocystis carinii* pneumonia and use of aerosolized pentamidine are particularly notable risk factors for pneumothorax.

Management

Patients with a small new pneumothorax should be **placed on 100% oxygen.** Small pneumothoraces often resolve spontaneously but may progress unpredictably to **tension pneumothorax,** which is treated by immediate insertion of a large-bore needle in the affected side. Patients with tension or secondary pneumothorax, those with severe symptoms, or those with a large pneumothorax should undergo **chest tube placement** (tube thoracostomy). Patients should be advised to **stop smoking,** because the risk of recurrence is 50% in patients who smoke. High altitudes, flying in unpressurized aircraft, and scuba diving should also be avoided. Thoracoscopy or open thoracotomy with stapling or laser pleurodesis is indicated with recurrent spontaneous pneumothorax, any bilateral pneumothorax, or failure of tube thoracostomy. Scarification by abrasion of the pleural surface may produce pleural symphysis.

Complications

Approximately 30% of patients with spontaneous pneumothorax develop recurrent episodes regardless of initial therapy (observation versus tube thoracostomy). Spontaneous pneumothorax may be complicated by **pneumomediastinum or subcutaneous emphysema.** Tension pneumothorax may be complicated by acute respiratory failure, cardiopulmonary arrest, or death.

Breakout Point

- Acute chest pain and dyspnea
- Primary spontaneous pneumothorax: tall, thin, healthy men with pleural blebs
- Secondary spontaneous pneumothorax: associated with COPD or underlying lung disease

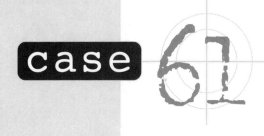

case 61

ID/CC	A **63-year-old woman** presents with **shortness of breath** and **sudden onset of chest pain.**
HPI	She was diagnosed with **carcinoma** of the colon 2 years ago. She complains of pain and swelling in her leg.
PE	VS: **tachypnea, tachycardia.** PE: **rales** in the right lung base; sternum and ribs are nontender; accentuated S_2.
Labs	CBC: normal. PT, PTT: normal. Factor V, protein C, protein S: normal.
Imaging	CTA, chest: **large filling defect in the right pulmonary artery.**

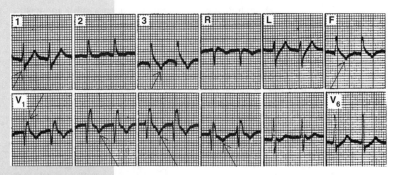

Figure 61-1. ECG: *arrows* indicate rightward axis shift in lead I; inverted T waves in leads III, aVF, V2–V4; prominent R wave of right bundle branch block in lead V1, all signs of right heart strain. Also note classic S1Q3T3 (large & wave in lead I, Q wave in lead III, inverted T wave in lead III).

case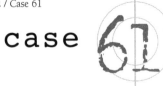

Pulmonary Embolus

Pathogenesis

Pulmonary embolus (PE) is a very dangerous and common complication of DVT in the lower extremities. Factors such as **pregnancy, OCP use, sepsis, surgery, DM, smoking, obesity, and immobilization** increase the risk of thrombosis and PE. The **classic triad of hemoptysis, dyspnea, and chest pain** actually occurs only in approximately 20% of patients with PE but tachynea and tachycardia are common. PE is known as the great pretender, because it may be asymptomatic or may present as chest pleurisy or discomfort. Massive PE may cause hypotension and right heart strain due to acute cor pulmonale.

Epidemiology

Very common cause of unexpected death, with 500,000 to 1 million cases per year. **PE occurs with increasing age, hypercoagulable states, underlying illness, and immobility.**

Management

Treatment of thromboembolism associated with a hypercoagulable state is 2-fold: acute and chronic therapy. Acutely, the clot may be lysed if it is life-threatening, by **thrombolytic agents (tPA and urokinase)**. If the clot is not life threatening, therapy with **heparin** to stabilize the clot is indicated. Following the treatment of the acute clot, chronic anticoagulant therapy must be initiated with either **warfarin (Coumadin) or low-molecular-weight heparin.** The question of whether to initiate prophylactic anticoagulation is based on the severity of initial presentation and risk factors related to subsequent clots.

Complications

Stroke, heart attack, and recurrent unexplained miscarriage or abortion.

Breakout Point

Risk Factors for Thromboembolism
• OCPs
• Pregnancy
• Sepsis
• DM
• Surgery
• Immobility
• Obesity
• Smoking

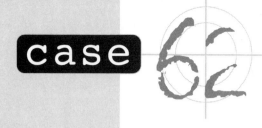

case 62

ID/CC	A **40-year-old African-American woman** complains of progressive **dyspnea on exertion, cough, chest discomfort, weight loss,** and loss of appetite.
HPI	The patient also complains of a purplish rash over her face. Her symptoms have progressed over the past year. She is a **nonsmoker.**
PE	VS: low-grade fever (38.2°C); tachypnea. PE: mild **respiratory distress; bluish-purple, swollen lesions** on nose, cheeks, and earlobes (LUPUS PERNIO); clubbing; bilateral fine inspiratory crackles.
Labs	CBC: lymphopenia. ESR elevated; **hypercalcemia; hyperglobulinemia;** serum **ACE levels elevated.** UA: 24-hour urine calcium elevated. Skin and transbronchial lung biopsies reveal **noncaseating granulomas;** staining and cultures negative for organisms. PFTs: reduced DL_{CO}; reduced FEV_1 and FVC; FEV_1/FVC ratio normal (**restrictive pattern of disease**); **Kveim–Siltzbach test** (antigen from human sarcoid tissue injected intradermally) positive.
Imaging	CXR: **bilateral hilar lymphadenopathy.**

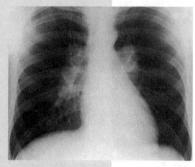

Figure 62-1. CXR: bilateral hilar lymphadenopathy.

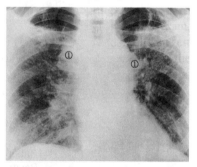

Figure 62-2. Later stage of lymphadenopathy (1) and reticulonodular densities. HRCT: presence of lymphadenopathy and pulmonary fibrosis confirmed. Nuc: gallium-67 lung scan positive (demonstrates diffuse uptake).

case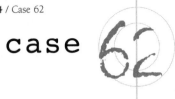

Sarcoidosis

Pathogenesis

The etiology of sarcoidosis is unknown. Accumulation of T cells, macrophages, and noncaseating granulomas in affected organs are seen, probably secondary to an exaggerated immune response to self-antigens or persistent foreign antigens. Organs most commonly affected are the **lungs, skin, eye, and lymph nodes.**

Epidemiology

Sarcoidosis occurs worldwide but is 10 times more prevalent and severe among **blacks** than among whites. Individuals 20 to 40 years of age are most often affected, with a slightly higher prevalence found among females. It is more common in **temperate climates** than in tropical zones and has a higher incidence among **nonsmokers.**

Management

Most patients are asymptomatic or undergo spontaneous remission within 2 years. Use **corticosteroids** for symptomatic pulmonary involvement, systemic symptoms, hypercalcemia, or involvement of extrapulmonary tissues that leads to organ dysfunction, iritis, and CNS and cardiac involvement. **Immunosuppressants** (eg, methotrexate, azathioprine) may be effective. Regular clinical evaluation is required.

Complications

Neurologic (peripheral neuropathy, cranial nerve palsies, papilledema, meningitis, epilepsy, cerebellar ataxia), cardiac (arrhythmias, CHF, cardiomyopathy), and ocular (anterior or posterior uveitis) manifestations may occur. Hypopituitarism, arthritis, cor pulmonale, and nephrocalcinosis occur as well.

Breakout Point

- Multiorgan disease
- "Potato nodules" in lung (bilateral hilar lymphadenopathy)
- Hypercalcemia, elevated ACE levels, noncaseating granulomas
- Erythema nodosum is the most common skin manifestation

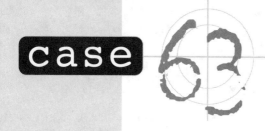

case 63

ID/CC A **52-year-old man** presents with increasing **shortness of breath on exertion.**

HPI The patient's medical history includes no cardiac or pulmonary disease. He has been working in the **stonecutting** industry for more than 25 years. His dyspnea on exertion has progressed over many years, and he denies any smoking, alcohol use, or illicit drug use. His family history is unremarkable.

PE VS: normal. PE: well developed and in no acute distress; no JVD, carotid bruits, or lymphadenopathy; **fine inspiratory crackles at the bases of lungs bilaterally;** cardiac exam normal with no extra heart sounds or murmurs; extremities notable only for **digital clubbing;** no cyanosis or edema.

Labs PFTs: mild obstructive and restrictive disease and decreased DL_{CO}.

Imaging CXR: diffuse ground-glass, nodular infiltrates with small, rounded opacities (silicotic nodules) throughout the lung; **peripheral calcifications in hilar lymph nodes** ("EGGSHELL CALCIFICATIONS") may be noted.

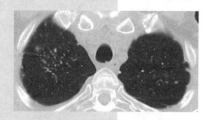

Figure 63-1. HRCT, chest: multiple small nodules are coalescing on the right side.

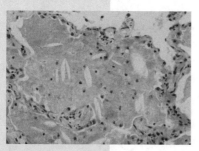

Figure 63-2. Pulmonary nodule is composed of refractile particles.

125

case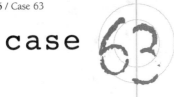

Silicosis

Pathogenesis

Silicosis represents a **diffuse fibrotic reaction of the lungs to inhalation of free crystalline silica particles that are ingested by alveolar macrophages, which rupture and subsequently release cytotoxic enzymes.** The silica is reingested by other macrophages, continuing a cycle of cytotoxic enzyme release and progressive local fibrotic reactions, ultimately producing acellular fibrous nodules characteristic of the clinical disease. Long-term exposure over 15 to 20 years results in **fibrosis** that is sufficient to produce characteristic small, rounded opacities in the upper lobes with retraction, hilar adenopathy, and "eggshell calcifications."

Epidemiology

Exposure to free silica or crystalline quartz occurs through major **occupational hazards such as rock mining, stonecutting, foundry work, quarrying (especially granite), tunneling, sandblasting, pottery-making, and packing of silica flour.** Progressive pulmonary fibrosis occurs in a dose-response fashion after many years. However, individuals working in small spaces can develop silicosis following periods of exposure as limited as 10 months.

Management

Cessation of silica exposure often necessitates a change in occupation. **Corticosteroids** may improve the chronic lymphocytic alveolitis. Screen for TB with tuberculin skin test and CXR, because patients with silicosis are clearly at **greater risk of acquiring** *Mycobacterium tuberculosis* (silicotuberculosis) as well as atypical mycobacterial infections. Multidrug treatment is indicated for any patient with a positive tuberculin test or old, healed tuberculous scars on CXR.

Complications

Progressive fibrosis may lead to coalescence of large irregular masses exceeding 1 cm in diameter (progressive massive fibrosis), leading to significant functional impairment with severe **restrictive and obstructive disease** on PFTs. Respiratory failure may follow within a few years. Atypical silicates such as talc may cause **pleural or lung cancers.**

Breakout Point

- Increases risk of TB
- "Eggshell calcifications" on CXR

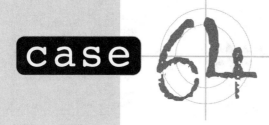

ID/CC A **21-year-old man** complains of **low back pain** and **stiffness**.

HPI He states that the pain is associated with **morning stiffness** that gradually **improves with exercise**. He also complains of **fatigue, weight loss,** and hip and shoulder pain.

PE VS: low-grade fever. PE: pallor; **stooped posture; reduced inspiratory chest excursion; high-pitched, blowing diastolic murmur** (aortic insufficiency); prominent abdomen; fixed kyphosis; **poor lumbar spinal mobility; loss of lumbar lordosis; sacroiliac joint tenderness.**

Labs CBC: anemia (Hct 30%). Low serum iron and TIBC (anemia of chronic disease); elevated ESR and C-reactive protein; elevated IgA; **negative RF and ANA**; positive **HLA-B27**.

Imaging XR: **periarticular sclerosis** with blurred sacroiliac joint margins.

RHEUMATOLOGY

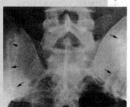

Figure 64-1. XR: **periarticular sclerosis** with blurred sacroiliac joint margins.

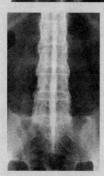

Figure 64-2. XR, spine: ankylosis and fusion of spinal vertebral bodies (BAMBOO SPINE) and sacroiliac joints.

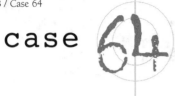

case

Ankylosing Spondylitis

Pathogenesis

AS is characterized by the presence of **inflammatory arthritis** of the **axial skeleton** (classically **sacroiliitis**) that may be accompanied by **peripheral arthritis, enthesitis** (inflammation at the site of tendinous or ligamentous attachment to bone), recurrent acute anterior **uveitis, aortic valve incompetence,** or pulmonary fibrosis. The precise etiology is unknown, but **immune-mediated mechanisms** are likely given the close association with HLA-B27, elevated serum levels of IgA and acute phase reactants, and an inflammatory histology. There is a significant association of AS with inflammatory bowel disease.

Epidemiology

AS usually begins in the second to third decade, is three times more common in **males** than in females, and is more prevalent among first-degree relatives who inherit the B27 allele.

Management

NSAIDs (eg, indomethacin) are the first line of therapy. Patients must **eliminate cigarette smoking,** initiate a **physical therapy** and **exercise** regimen, receive **genetic counseling,** and minimize spinal trauma to prevent fractures. Anti-TNF drugs (eg, etanercept or infliximab) are useful in the management of refractory cases. Other immunosuppressants and corticosteroids are of limited or no utility.

Complications

Complications include **spinal fractures and spondylodiscitis** after minimal trauma as well as **hip and knee deterioration** necessitating hip or knee replacement. Patients with long-standing disease may develop **aortic insufficiency, conduction defects,** deteriorating vision secondary to recurrent **uveitis** (40% of cases), pulmonary fibrosis, or chronic prostatitis.

Breakout Point

- Chronic low back pain in young adults
- Associated arthritis and uveitis
- Bamboo spine and blurred sacroiliac joint margins
- HLA-B27 positive

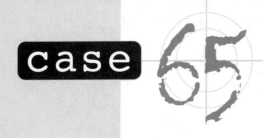

ID/CC A **45-year-old woman** complains of chronic progressive **muscle weakness** and **tenderness** associated with a diffuse **rash.**

HPI She is now unable to get up from a sitting position and also has **difficulty raising her arms and climbing stairs** (proximal muscle weakness). She also complains of difficulty swallowing (DYSPHAGIA).

PE PE: diffuse erythema over the face, neck, shoulders, and upper chest/back (SHAWL SIGN) and maculopapular eruptions; scaly patches over dorsum of PIP and metacarpal joints (GOTTRON SIGN); **lilac-colored** rash on eyelids (HELIOTROPE) with periorbital edema; decreased strength in proximal muscle groups.

Labs Markedly **elevated CK; elevated aldolase;** elevated ESR. UA: myoglobinuria. EMG: low amplitude, short duration motor unit action potentials. Muscle biopsy shows **inflammation** and muscle fiber **necrosis.**

Imaging XR, soft tissues: diffuse soft tissue calcifications.

RHEUMATOLOGY

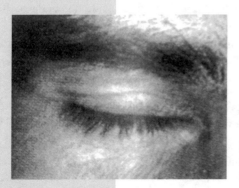

Figure 65-1. Lilac-colored rash on eyelids (HELIOTROPE) with periorbital edema.

case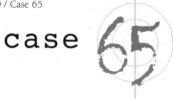

Dermatomyositis

Pathogenesis

Dermatomyositis is characterized by the presence of **polymyositis** in association with characteristic **skin changes.** Profound proximal muscle weakness, dysphagia, **respiratory impairment,** and **myocarditis** are key characteristics. The precise etiology is unknown, although viral infection, genetic factors, and autoimmunity are thought to be contributory mechanisms. Polymyositis/dermatomyositis may occur in **association with neoplasia** (breast, gynecologic, or rectal), vasculitis, or other connective tissue diseases (usually progressive systemic sclerosis, RA, mixed connective tissue disease, and SLE).

Epidemiology

May develop at any age, with a peak incidence between the fifth and sixth decades of life; **females outnumber males** by a ratio of 2 to 1. The 5-year survival rate is approximately 75%. Poor prognostic factors include delayed treatment, severe disease at initial presentation, underlying malignancy, associated connective tissue diseases, and the presence of antibodies to Jo-1 and signal recognition peptide.

Management

Corticosteroids are first-line agents, with improvement beginning as early as 1 to 4 weeks following the initiation of treatment. Measure progress with **serum enzymes. Cytotoxic drugs** (cyclophosphamide, methotrexate, and cyclosporine) may be used in refractory disease. Strength exercises and physical therapy are critical once control of the disease process is established.

Complications

Death may result from cardiac, pulmonary, or renal complications. Patients may have persistent muscle weakness, atrophy, or contracture.

Breakout Point

- Difficulty getting up from a chair or going up stairs
- Gottron papules and heliotrope rash
- Elevated CK
- No ocular or facial weakness (versus myasthenia gravis)

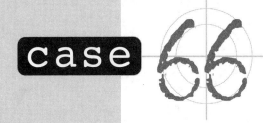

ID/CC A **45-year-old man** presents to the clinic complaining of **severe pain in the right big toe.**

HPI He states that he has had similar attacks in the past, each of which came on suddenly.

PE VS: low-grade fever (38.3 °C). PE: **tophi** in helix of ear and in hands and feet; **olecranon bursitis** bilaterally; **exquisitely tender, erythematous, swollen, shiny, and warm right first MTP joint** (PODAGRA).

Labs Serum **uric acid elevated**; synovial fluid aspiration reveals **negatively birefringent crystals** and elevated WBC (20,000).

Imaging XR foot: **punched-out erosions of bone** surrounded by cortical bone at the **MTP joint of the big toe.** XR, hand: soft tissue swelling (due to tophus) of the PIP joint of the index finger.

RHEUMATOLOGY

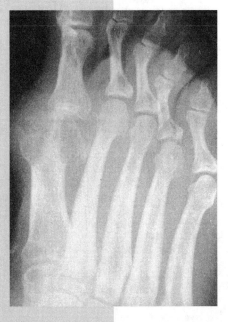

Figure 66-1. XR foot: punched-out erosions of bone surrounded by cortical bone at the MTP joint of the big toe.

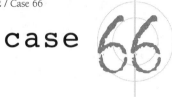

case 66

Gout

Pathogenesis

Gout is characterized by the presence of hyperuricemia with result-ant **arthritis** (usually monoarticular/inflammatory and presenting as repetitive acute episodes), **tophaceous deposition** in peri- and intra-articular locations, **urate nephropathy** (due to urate crystal deposition in interstitial renal parenchyma), and **nephrolithiasis.** Hyperuricemia may result from **increased dietary intake** of purines in foods **increased de novo synthesis** of purines due to increased activity of PRPP synthetase enzyme; increased breakdown of purines into uric acid due to a **deficiency of HGPRT**-mediated nucleotide salvage mechanism, as in Lesch–Nyhan syndrome; **accelerated purine nucleotide degradation** associated with conditions of rapid cell turnover (tumor lysis syndrome, myeloproliferative diseases, hemolysis, or rhabdomyolysis); or **undersecretion** (most individu-als with gout have **defective uric acid clearance).** In acute gout, ele-vated uric acid levels lead to the development of microtophi, which are shed into the joint space and are subsequently coated by immunoglobulins and complement, promoting phagocytosis by neutrophils. The crystals disrupt the phagosomal membranes, caus-ing lysosomal enzyme release into the joint space and enhancing inflammation.

Epidemiology

Gout arises primarily in **middle-aged and elderly men,** in **post-menopausal women,** and in patients with **end-stage renal disease.** Gout is seen more frequently with obesity, DM, hypertension, type II and type IV hyperlipidemia, and atherosclerosis. Additionally, gout may be precipitated by surgery, illness, or excessive alcohol consumption.

Management

Colchicine, NSAIDs, or **intra-articular glucocorticoids** for acute attacks. Use **allopurinol prophylaxis and uricosuric drugs (probenecid)** for chronic hyperuricemia. Encourage patients to avoid alcohol (inhibits urate excretion) and foods high in purines (eg, shellfish).

Complications

Nephrolithiasis, renal impairment, destructive arthropathy, and GI bleeding (secondary to high-dose NSAIDs).

Breakout Point

- Acute pain in MTP joint of big toe
- Urate crystals or tophi in joints is diagnostic
- Colchicine for acute attacks
- Allopurinol for chronic prophylaxis

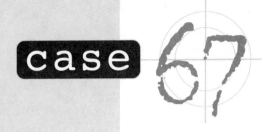

ID/CC A **67-year-old woman** presents with **pain in her knees and right shoulder** for the past 6 months.

HPI She reports the pain is **exacerbated with walking and relieved by rest,** with **no deformities or redness** over the knee joints. She thinks that her normal activity level is limited due to her knee and shoulder pain. She has no history of trauma and feels well.

PE VS: normal. PE: **crepitus** in both knees with full range of motion on active and passive movement, no knee effusion, no erythema, no edema bilaterally; normal gait.

Labs CBC normal.

Imaging XR, shoulder: **narrowing of joint space, osteophyte formation, thickened subchondral bone, bony cysts.** XR, knees: similar findings.

RHEUMATOLOGY

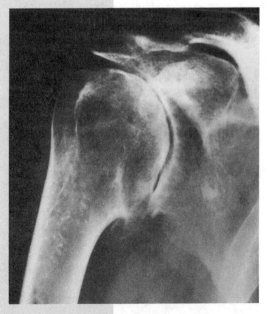

Figure 67-1. XR, shoulder: narrowing of joint space, osteophyte formation, thickened subchondral bone, bony cysts.

133

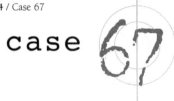

case

Osteoarthritis

Pathogenesis

Osteoarthritis is the **most common form of degenerative joint disease,** associated with **aging.** Etiology is **"wear and tear"** or wearing down of the articular cartilage over years of use. **Lack of systemic manifestations** and **lack of joint inflammation** are characteristic of this condition. Joints affected include weight-bearing joints such as the **knees or hips.** In the hands, only the **DIP and PIP** joints are affected. This contrasts with rheumatoid arthritis, which involves the wrist and MCP joints and spares the DIP joints.

Epidemiology

Osteoarthritis is present in 80%–90% of individuals older than 60 years of age.

Management

For mild disease, acetaminophen is recommended; for more severe disease, **NSAIDs** may be used. High-dose NSAID use is not needed, because this is not an inflammatory disorder. **Corticosteroid injections** may be performed up to four times per year. Surgical options of total hip or total knee replacements are available.

Complications

Presence in the knee is the leading cause of disability in the United States; presence in the back is a frequent cause of missed work.

Breakout Point

- "Wear and tear" arthritis
- Associated with aging
- Lack of joint inflammation

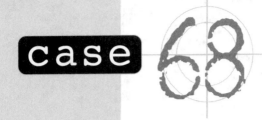

case 68

ID/CC	A **52-year-old man** complains of **weight loss, malaise,** fatigue, headache, and **muscle pain** of 6 months' duration.
HPI	He has no significant past medical history.
PE	VS: **fever** (38.5°C); hypertension (BP 178/95). PE: mild pallor; **diffuse palpable purpura and lacy reddish-blue rash on legs (livedo reticularis).**
Labs	CBC: anemia (Hct 33%); leukocytosis (13,000); **thrombocytosis;** no eosinophilia. Elevated ESR; hypergammaglobulinemia; **positive HBsAg.** UA: mild **proteinuria;** hematuria; **cellular casts.** Biopsy shows **necrotizing inflammation of small and medium-size arteries.**
Imaging	Angio, abdominal: **multiple aneurysms of small and medium-size blood vessels.**

RHEUMATOLOGY

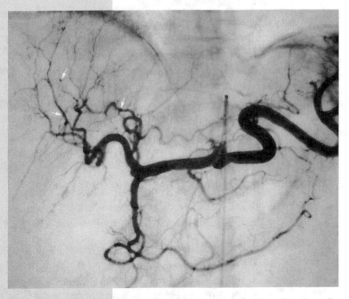

Figure 68-1. Angio, abdominal: multiple aneurysms of small and medium-size blood vessels.

case 68

Polyarteritis Nodosa

Pathogenesis

Polyarteritis nodosa is characterized by **necrotizing inflammation of small and medium-sized** arteries (such as renal and visceral arteries). **PMN infiltrates** are prevalent in the **acute stage** of the disease, whereas **mononuclear infiltrates** mark the **chronic stage** of illness. Fibrinoid necrosis later compromises the lumen, causing aneurysmal dilatation, thrombosis, and subsequent infarction of the tissues. Clinical manifestations indicate the organ system involvement: glomerular arteriolitis may present as hypertension and azotemia; vasa nervorum (arteries supplying nerves) involvement may present as **mononeuritis multiplex** (painful asymmetric motor and sensory neuropathy); and cardiac involvement may present as MI or CHF. The frequent presence of **Hepatitis B virus** suggests an immunologic component.

Epidemiology

A relatively uncommon illness that **presents between the fourth and fifth decades** and affects males and females equally. Associations have been found with SLE, RA, HBV infection, hairy cell leukemia, and serous otitis media.

Management

Prednisone in combination with **cyclophosphamide** has been shown to be effective. Early initiation of treatment is key. The **control of hypertension** is critical for reducing the morbidity and mortality of cardiac, renal, and CNS complications.

Complications

Death usually results from renal failure, GI complications (bowel infarct), and cardiovascular manifestations. Untreated polyarteritis nodosa has a 100% mortality rate.

Breakout Point

- Medium-vessel arteritis
- 10% associated with Hepatitis B virus
- Common symptoms are constitutional
- May present with livedo reticularis and mononeuritis multiplex

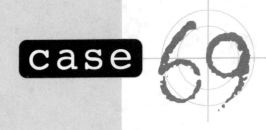

case 69

ID/CC A **70-year-old woman** presents with pain and **swelling in her right knee** that she has had for the past week.

HPI The pain has been **slowly progressive** over the past week and is so severe now that she cannot walk. She has had similar episodes in the past, which have affected her knees and wrists. She has a history of mild trauma to the knee a few years ago.

PE VS: normal. PE: knee is **warm, erythematous, edematous, diffusely tender** to light touch, range of passive and active motion limited due to pain, no crepitus; valgus, varus, anterior drawer test, posterior drawer test are negative; ballottement and milking show moderate knee effusion.

Labs Chem 10: normal. Joint fluid analysis: **WBC 50,000,** Gram stain negative, **rhomboid-shaped crystals.**

Imaging XR, knee: calcification of articular cartilage and soft tissues, and degenerative joint changes (osteoarthritis). Under red compensator light microscopy: **crystals are blue when parallel, yellow when perpendicular to the axis of the compensator.**

case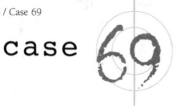

Pseudogout

Pathogenesis

Pseudogout is a crystal-induced arthropathy, characterized by the presence of **calcium pyrophosphate crystals** that show **positive birefringence under polarized light** (versus negatively birefringent crystals in gout). The etiology of crystal formation is unclear, but sequelae of pain and edema are due to infiltrating neutrophils and macrophages that release inflammatory cytokines. Joint involvement may be monoarticular or polyarticular, and is most common in the **knees,** followed by the wrists, elbows, shoulders, and ankles.

Epidemiology

Occurs equally in males and females, more commonly in patients 60 years of age or older.

Management

Treatment is supportive and directed at relief of pain and inflammation using **NSAIDs or steroids.** Unlike gout, there is no specific therapy to treat or prevent pseudogout attacks. Colchicine is not effective.

Complications

Recurrent injury associated with pseudogout predisposes the joint to increased incidence of infection.

Breakout Point

- Rhomboid-shaped crystals
- Positive birefringence under polarized light

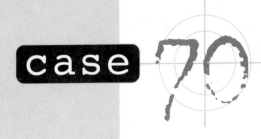

ID/CC A **36-year-old man** complains of **swelling and pain** in the **knee** and **ankle** that he has had for the past 2 weeks.

HPI He reports having suffered a severe case of *Salmonella* **enterocolitis** approximately 1 month ago. He also has **burning on urination** (due to urethritis), irritated eyes, occasional fever, and **moderate weight loss.**

PE VS: **fever** (38.6 °C). PE: mild clear, watery **conjunctival discharge**; mild **stomatitis**; tenderness to palpation, swelling, and erythema in knee and ankle with slight effusion.

Labs CBC/Lytes: normal. **ESR moderately elevated; RA factor negative**; synovial fluid culture negative; positive **HLA-B27.**

Imaging XR: permanent or progressive joint disease in peripheral joints (articular soft tissue swelling, joint space narrowing, marginal erosions) and in sacroiliac joints.

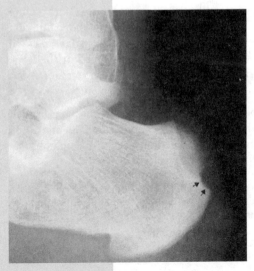

Figure 70-1. XR, ankle: striking bony erosion at the insertion of the Achilles tendon on the posterosuperior margin of the calcaneus.

case 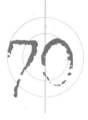 70

Reiter Syndrome

Pathogenesis

Reiter syndrome is characterized by the presence of **asymmetric "reactive arthritis"** (affecting large weight-bearing joints such as the knees and ankles or **sacroiliitis), conjunctivitis** or **uveitis, urethritis** (commonly a nongonococcal venereal infection), and **mucocutaneous lesions** (such as balanitis, stomatitis, and keratoderma blennorrhagicum). The presence of **HLA-B27** and characteristic XR findings are highly suggestive of the diagnosis of Reiter syndrome.

Epidemiology

Affects men and women equally following a dysenteric infection (*Salmonella, Shigella, Yersinia, Campylobacter*) or primarily males following an STD (*Chlamydia trachomatis* or *Ureaplasma urealyticum*) within the previous months. Classified as a form of reactive arthritis.

Management

NSAIDs for symptomatic relief. Use **corticosteroids** as needed. It is not known if antibiotics are effective in preventing this syndrome; however, it has been shown that prompt antibiotic administration for chlamydial urethritis may be beneficial. **Tetracycline** used for 3 months may reduce symptom duration and is particularly useful owing to its combination of antimicrobial and anti-inflammatory effects. **Sulfasalazine** is used for patients who are unresponsive to NSAIDs and antibiotic regimens.

Complications

Complications include urethral strictures, permanent joint damage, cataracts, carditis, aortic regurgitation, and **aortic root dissection.** Relapse is common.

Breakout Point

- Also called reactive arthritis
- 50%–80% are HLA-B27 positive
- Conjunctivitis, arthritis, urethritis, and mouth ulcers
- Occurs after dysentery or STD

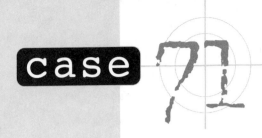

case 71

ID/CC A 45-year-old woman complains of **vague pain and stiffness** in her **wrists** and **hands** of several years' duration.

HPI Her pain is most **prominent in the morning,** with stiffness typically lasting for more than 30 minutes. She reports that her symptoms have progressed, as manifested by the formation of "bumps" (RHEUMATOID NODULES) on her **fingers, wrists,** and **elbows.** She additionally notes increased malaise, weight loss, and generalized weakness.

PE VS: normal. PE: extremities with decreased range of motion and swelling around **bilateral PIP and MCP joints;** flexion of DIP with extension of PIP (SWAN-NECK DEFORMITY); mild effusion and tenderness in both ankles; **ulnar deviation of digits at MCP joints with relative sparing of DIP joints;** subcutaneous nodules over bony prominences; hyperextension of DIP with flexion of PIP (BOUTONNIERE DEFORMITY); subcutaneous nodules on both elbows.

Labs CBC: normocytic, normochromic anemia; ESR moderately elevated; positive **RF;** elevated C-reactive protein; joint fluid with moderate elevation in WBC count (5,000–50,000/μL) and >50% PMNs on differential; negative culture.

Imaging See figures 71-1, 71-2, 71-3.

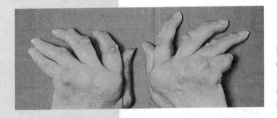

Figure 71-1. More advanced cases demonstrate arthritis mutilans, including ulnar deviation of the fingers and carpal fusion.

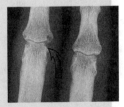

Figure 71-2. XR, hand: **periarticular osteoporosis** with **erosions** around the affected MCP and PIP joints.

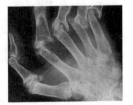

Figure 71-3. XR, hand: **periarticular osteoporosis** with **erosions** around the affected MCP and PIP joints.

case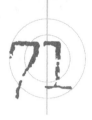

Rheumatoid Arthritis

Pathogenesis

RA is a chronic inflammatory disorder of **autoimmune** origin that is characterized by **synovitis of multiple joints with pannus formation.** Granulation tissue eventually erodes the cartilage, bone, ligaments, and tendons; scarring, contracture, and deformity result from inflammatory destruction of these structures. Any joint may be involved, but the **PIP, MCP, wrists, knees, ankles, and toes** are most commonly affected.

Epidemiology

RA is a common disease that **affects females three times more often than males.** The age of onset is usually 20 to 40 years, with prevalence increasing with age, although RA may present at any age. A strong association with **HLA-DR4** has been observed.

Management

Aspirins/NSAIDs are first-line therapy unless contraindicated. If these treatment modalities are unsuccessful, **immunosuppressive agents** such as methotrexate, gold salts, hydroxychloroquine, sulfasalazine, or azathioprine may be tried. TNF inhibitors may be used in patients who have not responded to methotrexate. Oral corticosteroids should be reserved for unresponsive cases, extra-articular disease or to relieve symptoms while waiting for the effect of immunosuppressive agents. Intra-articular corticosteroids may be tried when only one or two joints are inflamed. Key **nonpharmacologic measures** include weight loss, education, exercise, and assistive devices.

Complications

Complications include **atlantoaxial dislocation,** pleuropulmonary disease (**pleural effusion, pulmonary nodules, Caplan syndrome**), pericarditis, **Felty syndrome** (RA associated with splenomegaly and neutropenia), **vasculitis,** and pharmacologic therapy–related side effects (eg, aspirin/**NSAID-induced GI hemorrhage**). Factors associated with premature death include long length of disease, prolonged steroid use, early age at diagnosis, and low socioeconomic status.

Breakout Point

- Morning stiffness lasting more than 30 minutes
- Symmetric joint swelling with swan-neck deformities and boutonniere deformities
- Affects PIP, MCP, and wrists (spares the DIP joint)

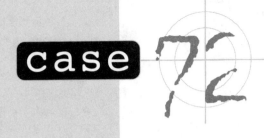
RHEUMATOLOGY

ID/CC A **45-year-old woman** presents with **joint aches** and **intermittent bluish tinge to her hands** that she has had for the past 2 months.

HPI She notes that the skin on her face and hands feels tight, has various areas of discoloration, and is itchy. Her hands turn blue and white when they are cold, and her fingertips seem to be peeling off. She has had difficulty swallowing both solids and liquids, with early satiety.

PE VS: normal. PE: skin exam shows alternating areas of **"salt and pepper" areas of hypo- and hyperpigmentation** on her face and hands; **telangiectasias** present on chest; ulcerations in fingertips (**calcinosis**); skin on face and hands is tight and shiny (can cause **sclerodactyly**); hands turn blue, white, and red when exposed to cold and subsequent warmth (**Raynaud phenomenon**).

Labs CBC: mildly anemic. **ANA positive with a speckled pattern. Anti-Scl-70 (against topoisomerase III), anticentromere antibody** (high specificity), **anti-RNAP (against RNA polymerases) positive.** ESR normal.

Imaging HRCT, chest: mild bibasilar pulmonary fibrosis. PFT: mild pulmonary hypertension. Esophagraphy: dysmotility and incompetent LES.

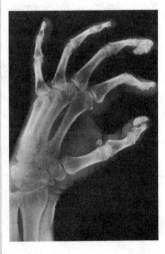

Figure 72-1. XR, hand: soft tissue calcifications in the distal phalanges.

case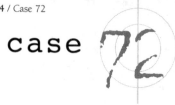

Scleroderma

Pathogenesis

Scleroderma (also called **systemic sclerosis**) encompasses heterogeneous diseases of two types: limited (80% of patients) and diffuse (20%). **CREST** syndrome is a type of limited scleroderma, characterized by **C**alcinosis cutis, **R**aynaud phenomenon, **E**sophageal dysmotility, **S**clerodactyly, **T**elangiectasias. The hallmark of scleroderma is fibrosis of skin and tissues. The etiology is unclear, but it is likely **autoimmune,** with activated fibroblasts, CD4 T cells, and monocyte infiltration in tissues.

Epidemiology

Scleroderma affects 3–20 per million people in the United States, predominantly females (5:1 female-to-male ratio) from the ages of 30–60 years.

Management

Treatment is **supportive,** with no specific therapy for the underlying process. Raynaud phenomenon is present in 95% of patients and can be treated with calcium channel blocker **(nifedipine)** or losartan. Iloprost (prostacyclin analog) causes vasodilation and is used to facilitate healing of digital ulcers. Prevention of gastroesophageal reflux and esophagitis with proton pump inhibitors is important. Corticosteroids are not effective.

Complications

Limited scleroderma has a 9-year survival rate of 40%. Diffuse disease has a worse prognosis, due to renal, cardiac, or pulmonary failure.

Breakout Point

CREST
Calcinosis cutis
Raynaud phenomenon
Esophageal dysmotility
Sclerodactyly
Telangiectasias

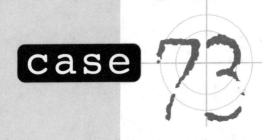

case 72

ID/CC A **34-year-old woman** presents to her physician with a **butterfly-shaped rash** over the bridge of her nose and cheeks that is **made worse by sunlight** (PHOTO-SENSITIVITY).

HPI The patient states that she has been experiencing increasing **malaise, fatigue, shortness of breath,** muscle aches, **joint pain,** swelling, and early-morning stiffness for the past 2 months.

PE VS: fever (38.9°C). PE: diffuse **maculopapular rash** over arms, back, and chest; raised, erythematous **malar rash** over cheeks and nose, extending to ears; **painless oral ulcers;** movements of knees, wrists, and joints of the hands are restricted and painful.

Labs CBC: normocytic, normochromic anemia; leukopenia. **ANA positive; elevated ESR; anti-Sm** and **anti-dsDNA antibodies** detected; serum C2, C4 complement factors decreased. UA: proteinuria; hematuria; cellular casts (due to lupus **nephritis**).

Imaging CXR: small right **pleural effusion.** Echo: no signs of pericarditis or pericardial effusion.

case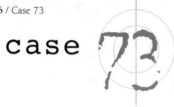

Systemic Lupus Erythematosus

Pathogenesis

SLE is an autoimmune disease of unknown etiology in which cells and tissues are damaged by **immune complexes** and **autoantibodies.** Lack of suppression by typical immunoregulatory systems produces **abnormal hyperactivity** of T and B cells. It is thought that genetic susceptibility, sex hormones, and exogenous antigens influence abnormal self-tolerance in these patients and promote immune cell activation. The antigens that stimulate autoantibodies are both **endogenous** and **exogenous.** Criteria for the diagnosis of SLE include **any four** of the following manifestations: malar rash; discoid rash; photosensitivity; oral ulcers; arthritis, serositis; ANAs; or renal, neurologic, hematologic, and immunologic disorders. The diagnosis of SLE can only be made after drug-induced lupus syndrome has been ruled out.

Epidemiology

90% of patients with SLE are **women,** typically of **childbearing years.** However, men, children, and the elderly can be affected. Prevalence is higher among **African Americans.** Sex hormones are thought to influence immune tolerance.

Management

Complete remission of SLE is rare. Patients with arthritis, mild pleurisy, and mild pericarditis should be treated with NSAIDs only. Use **antimalarial** drugs (retinal damage should be monitored) or **low-dose corticosteroids** for skin and musculoskeletal involvement. Life-threatening or severe SLE should be treated with **high-dose corticosteroids; cytotoxic agents** such as azathioprine, chlorambucil, and cyclophosphamide are useful for suppression of active disease and lowering the quantity of steroids needed.

Complications

Complications include **vasculitic lesions,** including purpura, ulcers, urticaria, and gangrene of the digits; **lupus nephritis;** cognitive dysfunction and seizures with **CNS complications;** ARDS and intra-alveolar hemorrhage; and pancreatitis, abdominal discomfort, diarrhea, vasculitis, and peritonitis. Pericarditis, myocarditis, effusions, arrhythmias, and infarction are manifestations of **cardiac lupus; pleural effusions** may lead to atelectasis, pneumonitis, and infection.

Breakout Point

- Occurs in young women
- Butterfly rash over face
- Multisystem autoimmune disease
- Anti-Smith, Anti-dsDNA, and ANA positive

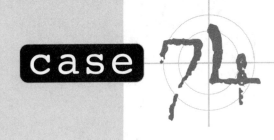

ID/CC A **24-year-old woman** presents with **fever, fatigue, joint aches, and blurred vision** of 2 months' duration.

HPI She reports intercurrent episodes of **headaches, dizziness, fatigue, myalgias, chest pain, and lethargy.** She has tried multiple over-the-counter cold medications, completed courses of antibiotics, and tried antidepressants as an outpatient with persistence of symptoms. She recently underwent MR imaging of the head, which was negative. She is up-to-date on vaccinations and had been previously healthy.

PE VS: **BP 140/60 in right arm, 100/40 in left arm**. PE: thin Asian female; **carotid bruits** with rapid upstrokes; **diminished pulses in upper extremities.**

Labs CBC: leukocytosis, normochromic normocytic anemia, thrombocytosis. ANA negative. ESR elevated.

Imaging MR and T2-weighted images of the chest: aortic thickening, edema in the aorta wall, with luminal narrowing. **Arteriography: aortic arch vessels have areas of occlusion and aneurysms.**

RHEUMATOLOGY

case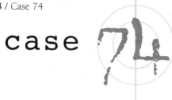

Takayasu Arteritis

Pathogenesis

Takayasu arteritis (**pulseless disease**) is a rare vasculitis with predilection for the aortic arch vessels. The etiology is unknown. Monocytic infiltration, transmural granulomatous inflammation, and fibrosis causes stenoses, occlusions, and aneurysms. Typical findings include diminished peripheral pulses, asymmetric blood pressure measurements, and vascular bruits.

Epidemiology

Rare, affects approximately 1–3 individuals per million in the United States, and most commonly occurs in Asian females younger than 40 years of age.

Management

Prednisone is effective during the early "inflammatory" stage in limiting progression. Stenoses can be treated with percutaneous **angioplasty or stenting**, although there is a high recurrence rate. Surgery (bypass of stenosed segments) is reserved for late and resistant occlusive disease.

Complications

These are related to ischemia from occlusive disease and include TIAs, stroke, and angina from chronic aortic dissection.

Breakout Point

- Pulseless disease
- Asymmetric BP measurements
- Affects aortic arch vessels
- Young Asian females

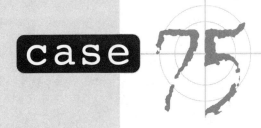

case 75

ID/CC A **42-year-old Caucasian woman** presents with increasing **sinus pain, bloody nasal discharge**, and **difficulty breathing.**

HPI The patient adds that she has been experiencing **hemoptysis, shortness of breath,** and general chest discomfort. She also complains of increasing malaise, weakness, loss of appetite, and weight loss.

PE VS: low-grade fever (38.1 °C); tachypnea (RR 24). PE: episcleritis; nasal mucosa ulcerated with bloody discharge; coarse breath sounds bilaterally.

Labs CBC: leukocytosis and mild anemia. **ESR markedly elevated; antineutrophil cytoplasmic antibodies** (ANCAs; C-ANCA more specific) present; biopsy of lung lesion reveals necrotizing granulomatous vasculitis. UA: **proteinuria** and **hematuria (secondary to glomerulonephritis).**

Imaging CXR: cavitating nodules.

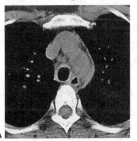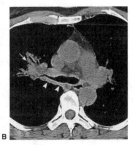

Figure 75-1. CT, chest **(A)** Circumferential thickening of tracheal wall. **(B)** Thickening of right main bronchus and right upper lobe bronchus with narrowing of airway lumen (*arrow*).

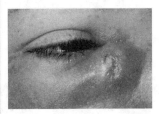

Figure 75-2. Inflammation of sinuses.

RHEUMATOLOGY

149

case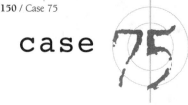

Wegener Granulomatosis

Pathogenesis

WG is characterized by **granulomatous vasculitis** of the **upper and lower respiratory tracts** with **glomerulonephritis**. Lung involvement appears as multiple, nodular cavitary infiltrates. Upper airway lesions, especially in the sinuses, demonstrate necrosis, inflammation, and granulomas formation.

Epidemiology

WG is a rare disease that affects men and women equally. The disease rarely affects patients before adolescence; mean age of onset is 40 years.

Management

The treatment of choice is **cyclophosphamide** given in combination with **steroids**. WBC count and renal function should be closely monitored. Remissions can be induced in most patients; long-term follow-up is required.

Complications

Focal and segmental glomerulitis may progress into a **rapidly progressive crescentic glomerulonephritis**; nasal ulceration may produce **septal perforation** that may result in **saddle-nose deformity**. Eye complications can produce episcleritis, scleritis, and sclerouveitis.

Breakout Point

- Triad of upper respiratory tract disease, lower respiratory tract disease, and glomerulonephritis
- Presents as sinusitis refractory to treatment
- Renal disease may rapidly progress
- ANCA-positive (c-ANCA more specific)

questions

1. A 63-year-old woman complains of pain in her fingers along with stiffness that is worse when she wakes up in the morning and improves as the day progresses. On exam, all of her fingers display prominent swan-neck deformities as well as boutonniere deformities. Her family physician had placed her on NSAIDs for years; however, she developed an upper GI bleed with evidence of an ulcer in her gastric fundus. She is referred to a rheumatologist for treatment recommendations. Which of the following is the most reasonable treatment alternative?

   A. Oral prednisone
   B. Intra-articular steroid injections
   C. Etanercept
   D. Methotrexate
   E. Rituximab

2. A 21-year-old male college soccer player is brought to the ER with complaints of extreme shortness of breath that brought him to his knees during a game he was playing. He also complains of severe pain in the right hemithorax. On exam, he is a tall slim male in moderate distress. He has greatly diminished breath sounds over the right lung fields. His pulse oximetry is 85%. Which of the following is the most reasonable first step after the patient is placed on supplemental oxygen?

   A. Obtain a portable CXR
   B. Request a V/Q scan
   C. Perform a CT scan of the chest
   D. Insert a large-bore needle in the affected side
   E. Place a chest tube

3. A 65-year-old woman suffers from multiple medical conditions, including peripheral vascular disease, CAD, neuropathy, and end-stage renal disease as a result of years of poorly controlled DM. She reports to the dialysis center where routine laboratory studies are taken. Her potassium is 6.4 mEq/L. An ECG is performed, demonstrating peaked T waves. Which of the following is the appropriate pharmacologic intervention?

A. Kayexalate
B. Metoprolol
C. Glucose and insulin
D. Calcium gluconate
E. Spironolactone

4. A 43-year-old African-American woman complains to her family physician of progressive shortness of breath and weight loss. A CXR demonstrates bilateral hilar adenopathy. Mediastinoscopy is performed, demonstrating final pathology consistent with noncaseating granulomas. A special stain for organisms returns negative, and a presumptive diagnosis of sarcoidosis is rendered. Which of the following is an additional expected finding?

A. Increased DL_{CO}
B. Increased FEV_1
C. Decreased FEV_1/FVC ratio
D. Decreased FVC
E. Decreased serum calcium

5. A 62-year-old man presents to the pulmonologist with complaints of progressive shortness of breath and dyspnea on exertion. He admits to a 90-pack-year history of tobacco use. On exam, he appears in mild distress and has difficulty completing a sentence without stopping for a breath. As well, he is quite barrel-chested with distant breath sounds, and his lungs are hyperresonant to percussion. He denies any significant family history of lung disease. Which of the following is the most likely diagnosis?

A. Paraseptal emphysema
B. Panacinar emphysema
C. Chronic bronchitis
D. Centriacinar emphysema
E. Alpha-1 antitrypsin deficiency

6. A 24-year-old woman presents to a family physician with complaints of malaise, weakness, and a persistent headache. A physical exam reveals a well-developed female in no acute distress with a loud epigastric bruit. She is referred for renal artery angiography, which demonstrates a "string of beads" appearance of the right renal artery. Which of the following offers the best chance of "cure" for this patient's condition?

A. Right nephrectomy
B. Percutaneous transluminal angioplasty
C. Corticosteroids
D. ACE therapy
E. Angioembolization of the lesion

7. A 65-year-old man presents with progressive proximal muscle weakness manifested by difficulty rising from an arm chair and difficulty climbing up steps. He has a distinctive heliotropic rash involving the eyelids, as well as Groton lesions on his elbows and knees. A muscle biopsy confirms the diagnosis of dermatomyositis. Which of the following should be considered to complete his workup?

   A. Measurement of SS-A and SS-B autoantibodies
   B. Measurement of serum creatinine levels
   C. Measurement of anti-DNA topoisomerase antibody levels
   D. An EEG
   E. A CT scan of the chest, abdomen, and pelvis

8. A 17-year-old boy presents to his internist for a physical exam before going away to college. His only complaint is feeling short of breath, especially at night or when exercising. He notes this occurs more than twice a week and is often accompanied by a cough. He notes several environmental allergens. On exam, he has a prolonged expiratory wheeze. PFTs reveal a decreased FEV1/FVC ratio. Given his new diagnosis of asthma, which of the following is the most appropriate therapy?

   A. Short-acting adrenergic inhaler only
   B. Short-acting adrenergic inhaler plus low-dose inhaled steroids
   C. Short-acting adrenergic inhaler plus moderate-dose inhaled steroids
   D. High-dose inhaled steroids and long-acting adrenergic agonist
   E. Omalizumab (anti-IgE antibody)

9. A 30-year-old man presents to his physician with malaise, fever, cough, and myalgias over the last week. He tells his physician he is a landscaper for a prestigious golf club in Palm Springs and has been late to get the course ready for a nationally televised event. On exam, he has painful lesions over his shins. A positive *Coccidioides* skin test confirms a diagnosis of *Coccidioides immitis* infection. Which of the following skin lesions is associated with this condition also known as desert rheumatism?

   A. Psoriasis
   B. Molluscum contagiosum
   C. Seborrheic dermatitis
   D. Pityriasis versicolor
   E. Erythema nodosum

10. A 27-year-old male nursing aide presents to the employee health office with a painful vesicle grouping on his fingers. He notes that he has been changing the sheets of a patient with disseminated HSV infection and AIDS. The terminal phalange of the first four digits on his left hand have vesicular lesions, of which one is oozing fluid that is taken for testing. The sample demonstrates a positive Tzanck test. Which of the following is a likely diagnosis?

   A. Herpetic whitlow
   B. Herpes gladiatorum
   C. Dermatitis herpetiformis
   D. Kaposi sarcoma
   E. Herpes zoster

11. A 23-year-old college senior returns here after spring break in Mexico. He reports to his physician 2 weeks later with extreme fatigue, sore throat, and a low-grade fever. On exam, he has painless cervical adenopathy and swollen tonsils but no tonsillar exudates. His abdominal exam demonstrates a tender left upper quadrant. Which of the following would most likely reveal the suspected diagnosis?

   A. PBS
   B. Western blot
   C. Weil-Felix Test
   D. Stool sample for ova and parasites
   E. Elevated IgE levels

12. A 47-year-old Asian-American woman brings her mother to the family physician for complaints of fevers, night sweats, and blood-tinged sputum for the past 3 months, since coming to the United States from China. A CXR reveals a cavitary lesion in the right upper lobe. The patient is placed on a multidrug regimen for TB, because her sputum returns positive for acid fast bacilli. Which of the following represents the appropriate management of the patient's daughter?

   A. Administer a PPD, and if the induration is >15 mm, administer multidrug treatment
   B. Administer a PPD, and if the induration is >15 mm, administer rifampin
   C. Administer a PPD, and if the induration is >10 mm, administer INH
   D. Administer a PPD, and if the induration is >5 mm, administer BCG immunization
   E. Administer a PPD, and if the induration is >5 mm, administer INH

13. A 68-year-old woman presents to her family physician with complaints of generalized weakness. She has a history of long-standing diabetes with poor kidney function. Routine serum and urine chemistries are ordered, as well as ABGs. The results demonstrate hyperkalemia, hyperchloremia, and elevated BUN and creatinine, with a non–anion gap metabolic acidosis as well as an elevated uric acid with a positive urinary anion gap. Which of the following is the most likely cause of her metabolic derangement?

    A. Type I RTA
    B. Type II RTA
    C. Type III RTA
    D. Type IV RTA
    E. Excess mineralocorticoid production

14. A 22-year-old man is brought to the ER after being shot in the abdomen. He is taken to surgery, where it is found that his IVC was destroyed by the bullet, requiring ligation of the vessel below the renal vein. He required several units of blood. Now, 3 days later, his urine output has decreased significantly as reported on his ins/outs on the chart. Which of the following is the next step in the management of his decreasing urine output?

    A. Perform hemodialysis
    B. Administer isotonic saline intravenously
    C. Obtain laboratory tests to determine FE_{Na}
    D. Administer IV furosemide
    E. Administer dopamine

15. A 56-year-old woman visits her family physician because of lower extremity swelling as well as generalized edema. Her past medical history includes HBV, an unspecified heart arrhythmia managed with antiarrhythmics, uncontrolled hypertension, a history of Hodgkin disease, and a history of urinary sepsis requiring IV antibiotics. Laboratory tests demonstrate 3+ protein in her urine. She is referred to a nephrologist for a kidney biopsy, which demonstrates thickened GBMs with a "spike and dome" pattern. Immunofluorescence demonstrates granular deposits of IgG and C3 along capillary loops. Which of the following could have controlled her newly diagnosed kidney disease?

    A. Hepatitis B interferon
    B. The amiodarone used for the treatment of her arrhythmia
    C. The chemotherapy she receives for her Hodgkin lymphoma
    D. The hydralazine she takes to control her blood pressure
    E. The gentamicin she received while she was hospitalized for urosepsis

16. A 13-year-old boy notes numerous episodes of "pneumonia" growing up. Often he wakes up in the morning coughing up a half cup of purulent-appearing sputum. He has been referred to a pulmonologist at the request of his family physician, who has attempted to treat his respiratory infections with numerous antibiotics. The pulmonologist orders a CT scan of the chest that reveals honeycombing along the bronchioles. The boy's condition can be associated with which of the following disorders?

   A. Goodpasture syndrome
   B. Q fever
   C. Osler-Weber-Rendu disease
   D. Felty syndrome
   E. Kartagener syndrome

17. A 33-year-old HIV-positive man is brought by his partner to the ER. The companion notes that the patient has not been himself lately and that he has been "acting kind of weird." The patient does complain of both photophobia as well as phonophobia. A CT scan is performed, demonstrating a ring-enhancing mass in the frontal lobe. The patient has not been taking his HIV medications regularly. Which of the following is the most reasonable treatment to begin?

   A. Temozolomide
   B. Intrathecal methotrexate
   C. Pyrimethamine
   D. Dapsone and rifampin
   E. Intrathecal vancomycin

18. A 27-year-old woman reports to her family physician with complaints of malaise, a week-long low-grade fever, and fatigue. On exam, she has no detectable radial pulses bilaterally; however, femoral pulses are well appreciated. Laboratory results demonstrate an elevated ESR and CRP, but they are negative for anti-dsDNA antibodies. Vascular studies demonstrate severe stenosis of the branches of the aortic arch. Which of the following is the likely diagnosis?

   A. Polymyalgia rheumatica
   B. Kawasaki disease
   C. Behçet disease
   D. Sjögren syndrome
   E. Takayasu arteritis

19. A 56-year-old man presents to the internist with complaints of progressive shortness of breath with exertion. He denies any significant
tobacco use but admits to working in the concrete business for years
with significant dust exposure. On exam, he has fine inspiratory
crackles with prominent clubbing of his fingers. A CXR performed in
the office demonstrates egg-shell calcifications. Which of the following is the most logical step in the management of this patient's new
diagnosis?

A. Begin high-dose steroids
B. Place a PPD
C. Administer epinephrine
D. Obtain a pleural biopsy
E. Treat the patient for allergic bronchopulmonary aspergillosis

20. A mail clerk at the governor's office opens a piece of mail addressed
to the governor sent in an envelope with no return address. On open-
ing the letter a cloud of white dust arises from the envelope. Given
the recent scares on television, the worker immediately informs the
Federal Bureau of Investigation, who isolate the building.
Microbiologists in special containment suits are brought in to collect
samples. In the meantime, the patient develops a fever and ulcerative
lesions on his hands. Back at the laboratory, cultures are performed
yielding the identification of *Francisella tularensis*. Which of the following is true of this organism?

A. It can be directly spread between infected persons
B. A vaccine is available to the public
C. The lethality results from the pneumonic and typhoidal forms of
the diseases
D. Infection is associated with infected cattle
E. The drug of choice for the treatment is streptomycin.

answers

1-D

    A. Oral prednisone [incorrect]. Oral steroids should be used only in refractory cases of RA, when other alternatives have been exhausted. In addition, steroids interfere with prostaglandin synthesis that would contribute to GI ulceration.

    B. Intra-articular steroid injections [incorrect]. Although sometimes used when one or a few joints are involved, intra-articular steroids would not be used in the phalanges as in this case.

    C. Etanercept [incorrect]. TNF antagonists, such as Etanercept [incorrect], infliximab, and adalimumab are increasingly being used as monotherapy or as part of multidrug regimens. However, they are extremely expensive.

    D. Methotrexate [correct]. Methotrexate is one of the most popular disease-modifying antirheumatic drugs. It has good efficacy, a favorable toxicity profile, early onset of action, and relatively low cost.

    E. Rituximab [incorrect]. Rituximab, a recombinant anti-CD20 antibody, is used for the treatment of non-Hodgkin lymphoma. It has recently been approved in patients with RA who have not had an adequate response to anti-TNF agents.

2-D

    A. Obtain a portable CXR [incorrect]. In this case, a pneumothorax may be detected radiographically on a CXR, although the delay would result in increased respiratory distress and should be addressed urgently and empirically.

    B. Request a V/Q scan [incorrect]. A V/Q scan may demonstrate a pulmonary embolism; however, this is not a pulmonary embolism.

    C. Perform a CT scan of the chest [incorrect]. Although a CT scan can be used to detect a pneumothorax, this would introduce delay and is not a treatment.

    D. Insert a large-bore needle in the affected side [correct]. Placement of a large bore needle at the second or third intercostal space at the midaxillary line allows aspiration of the pneumothorax.

    E. Place a chest tube [incorrect]. Placement of a chest tube may be necessary if needle aspiration does not result in resolution of the pneumothorax.

3-D

A. Kayexalate [incorrect]. Kayexalate is a cation exchange resin that decreases serum potassium and causes diarrhea. It is used to decrease potassium levels in patients with mildly elevated levels without ECG changes.

B. Metoprolol [incorrect]. Beta$_2$-adrenergic agonists do have a role in the treatment of hypercalcemia, but metoprolol is a beta-antagonist.

C. Glucose and insulin [incorrect]. These substances are used to decrease potassium by driving extracellular potassium into the cells. They, however, are not the most immediate treatment of hyperkalemia in the face of ECG changes.

D. Calcium gluconate [correct]. This is indeed the initial drug given in symptomatic hyperkalemia. It serves to stabilize cardiac membranes and prevent fatal arrhythmias.

E. Spironolactone [incorrect]. Potassium-sparing diuretics, such as spironolactone contribute to hyperkalemia and are to be used with caution in kidney patients.

4-D

A. Increased DL_{CO} [incorrect]. The DL_{CO} is increased with large lung volumes or even in patients with asthma. However, patients with sarcoidosis have a decreased DL_{CO}.

B. Increased FEV_1 [incorrect]. Again, sarcoidosis is associated with a decrease in FEV_1. FEV_1 can however be increased in patients with asthma and treated with bronchodilators.

C. FEV_1/FVC ratio [incorrect], Patients with obstructive lung diseases have a decreased FEV_1/FVC ratio. However, sarcoidosis is a restrictive lung disease with a normal FEV_1/FVC ratio.

D. Decreased FVC [correct]. Sarcoidosis is indeed a restrictive lung disease and by definition has a decreased FVC. Patients with obstructive lung disease have normal or lightly decreased lung capacity.

E. Decreased serum calcium [incorrect]. Patients with sarcoidosis have hypercalcemia, not hypocalcemia, as well as elevated ACE levels.

5-D

A. Paraseptal emphysema [incorrect]. Paraseptal emphysema involves the distal portions of the respiratory unit adjacent to the pleura. This type of emphysema is thought to underlie many of the cases of spontaneous pneumothorax in young adults.

B. Panacinar emphysema [incorrect]. Panacinar emphysema involves the acini from the level of the respiratory bronchiole to the terminal alveoli. It is the type of emphysema most closely associated with alpha 1 anti-trypsin deficiency.

C. Chronic bronchitis [incorrect]. Chronic bronchitis is a distinct form of COPD associated with hyperplasia of mucous cells. This case does not describe such a patient.

D. Centriacinar emphysema [correct]. Centriacinar emphysema with involvement of the proximal portions of the acini and relative sparing of the distal portions is most closely associated with cigarette smoking. Cigarette smoking interferes with the enzymes such as elastase that are involved in normal lung remodeling.

E. Alpha-1 antitrypsin deficiency [incorrect]. This genetic disease is characterized by panacinar emphysema as well as liver cirrhosis.

6-B

A. Right nephrectomy [incorrect]. Because the disease is in the renal artery and not the kidney itself, a nephrectomy would be far too aggressive approach in the case of fibromuscular dysplasia.

B. Percutaneous transluminal angioplasty [correct]. This form of angioplasty, with successful stenting of the involved renal artery, results in resolution of the hypertension in greater than 50% of cases.

C. Corticosteroids [incorrect]. Although corticosteroids are used in the treatment of several arteritides, fibromuscular dysplasia results from intimal hyperplasia and not inflammation, so there is no role for steroids.

D. ACE therapy [incorrect]. ACE inhibitors do have a role in the medical management, because the hypertension is the result of activation of the renin–angiotensin–aldosterone axis by the kidney affected by the stenosis.

E. Angioembolization of the lesion [incorrect]. Angioembolization of the lesions in the kidney cells can be considered in patients with hemangiomas of the kidney with impending rupture or hemodynamic instability.

7-E

A. Measurement of SS-A and SS-B autoantibodies [incorrect]. SS-A and SS-B, also known as anti-Ro and anti-La, are antibodies against ribonucleoproteins that are elevated in Sjögren syndrome.

B. Measurement of serum creatinine levels [incorrect]. Although serum CK is elevated in polymyositis, the disease does not affect the kidney and there is no reason to assume the serum creatinine would be elevated.

C. Measurement of anti-DNA topoisomerase antibody levels [incorrect]. Antitopoisomerase antibodies (anti-SCL70) are more-or-less unique to the connective tissue disorder systemic sclerosis.

D. An EEG [incorrect]. Although EMG is helpful in the diagnosis of muscular conditions such as polymyositis, there is no role for an EEG.

E. A CT scan of the chest, abdomen, and pelvis [correct]. Dermato-myositis, a condition associated with anti-Jo-1 antibodies, is also considered with underlying malignancy in 6% to 45% of patients. Imaging to rule out malignancy such as CT of the chest, abdomen, and pelvis would be prudent.

8-B

A. Short-acting adrenergic inhaler only [incorrect]. The appropri-ate treatment for mild intermittent asthma, with symptoms less than twice per week, is a short-acting adrenergic inhaler alone.

B. Short-acting adrenergic inhaler plus low-dose inhaled steroids [correct]. This patient has mild persistent asthma with symp-toms more than twice per week. This requires the use of either leukotriene inhibitor or low-dose inhaled steroids along with a short-acting adrenergic inhaler.

C. Short-acting adrenergic inhaler plus moderate-dose inhaled steroids [incorrect]. This therapy is used to treat patients with symptoms that occur daily and interfere with activities (moder-ate persistent asthma).

D. High-dose inhaled steroids and long-acting adrenergic agonist [incorrect]. Patients with severe persistent asthma that interferes with daily living and limits activity are best managed with high-dose inhaled steroids with long-acting adrenergic agonists.

E. Omalizumab (anti-IgE antibody) [incorrect]. This recombinant anti-IgE antibody is approved for the treatment of moderate to severe persistent asthma whose symptoms are not adequately controlled with inhaled corticosteroids.

9-E

A. Psoriasis [incorrect]. Psoriasis is scaly salmon pink lesions on the extensor surfaces of the elbows and knees that can be asso-ciated with arthritis (psoriatic arthritis).

B. Molluscum contagiosum [incorrect]. Molluscum contagiosum is a dome-shaped fleshy papule with central umbilications due to a virus related to smallpox.

C. Seborrheic dermatitis [incorrect]. Greasy scales overlying erythematous plaques is a common description of seborrheic dermatitis commonly found on the scalp, eyebrows, eyelids, and nasolabial folds.

D. Pityriasis versicolor [incorrect].A common benign condition due to the superficial mycosis. *Malassezia furfur* manifests with hypopigmented and hyperpigmented macules on the chest and back.

E. Erythema nodosum [correct]. This skin condition is associated with several infectious agents, including coccidiomycosis as well as inflammatory conditions such as ulcerative colitis or even some drugs such as sulfonamides.

10-A

A. Herpetic whitlow [correct]. This occupational disease results from inoculations of HSV-infected body fluids via a break in the skin of health care workers. After the resolution of the primary infection, it resides in local ganglia and can reactivate.

B. Herpes gladiatorum [incorrect]. This affects wrestlers, judo players, or athletes in other sports where there is close contact between participants. Infection results from skin contact between infected individuals or the mats on which the events take place.

C. Dermatitis herpetiformis [incorrect]. This pruritic vesiculopapular rash is not associated with herpes infection; rather it is almost always associated with celiac disease (gluten-sensitive enteropathy).

D. Kaposi sarcoma [incorrect]. Kaposi sarcoma is associated with HIV infection. However, such lesions are not transmissible by contact.

E. Herpes zoster [incorrect]. This can cause severe life-threatening infections in immunocompromised patients, such as those with AIDS. However, again, it is unlikely to cause the lesion in health care workers even with contact.

11-A

A. PBS [correct]. A PBS in a patient with infectious mononucleosis displays at least 10% atypical lymphocytes.

B. Western blot [incorrect]. This test is used for the initial screening of HIV. Although many of the symptoms between HIV and mononucleosis overlap, HIV infection is usually associated as well with diarrhea, weight loss, nausea, and vomiting.

C. Weil-Felix test [incorrect]. Rickettsial infections such as epidemic typhus, characterized by influenza-like symptoms as well as a truncal rash are confirmed by the Weil-Felix test.

D. Stool sample for ova and parasites [incorrect]. Ova and parasites tests of stool are important to detect protozoal infections such as *Entamoeba histolytica,* which are endemic to countries such as Mexico. Fortunately, the patient has no complaints of diarrheal illness.

E. Elevated IgE levels [incorrect]. Although patients have elevated heterophile antibodies, these antibodies are IgM antibodies. Patients with asthma and other atopic conditions can have elevated IgE levels.

12-E

A. Administer a PPD, and if the induration is >15 mm, administer multidrug treatment [incorrect]. The threshold for treatment in patients in which the area of induration is 15 mm are those for low-risk patients, of which a contact of an active case is not.

B. Administer a PPD, and if the induration is >15 mm, administer rifampin [incorrect]. The correct prophylactic treatment for patients above a PPD cutoff appropriate for their risk is INH [incorrect].

C. Administer a PPD, and if the induration is >10 mm, administer INH [incorrect]. Patients who have a positive PPD threshold of 10 mm are those who are foreign-born, from low-income populations, IV drug users, residents of long-term care facilities, or homeless.

D. Administer a PPD, and if the induration is >5 mm, administer BCG immunization [incorrect]. BCG immunizations are used in countries outside the United States. It is an immunization from a live strain of mycobacterium related to *Mycobacterium tuberculosis.*

E. Administer a PPD, and if the induration is >5 mm, administer INH [correct]. The positive threshold for a PPD in immediate contacts with active disease is 5 mm. The correct prophylactic drug is INH, which could be administered with pyridoxine.

13-D

A. Type I RTA [incorrect]. Type I RTA is rather rare and results from deficient H^+ secretions in the distal tubules; the urine would not be so acidic.

B. Type II RTA [incorrect]. Type II RTA is quite rare and due to defective bicarbonate reabsorption in the proximal tubules. One would not expect hyperkalemia, rather hypokalemia.

C. Type III RTA [incorrect]. Currently, there is no type III RTA; it was formerly type I with a component of type II. Now this is considered a variant of type I RTA.

D. Type IV RTA [correct]. This is the most common form of RTA and presents with the derangements as illustrated in the case. It is associated with DM as well as interstitial nephritis.

E. Excess mineralocorticoid production [incorrect]. RTA results in part from a relative deficiency of the mineralocorticosteroids, and the treatment often entails the use of replacements such as fludrocortisone.

14-C

A. Perform hemodialysis [incorrect]. Hemodialysis is indicated only for severe hyperkalemia, pulmonary edema, refractory acidosis, pericarditis, uremia, encephalopathy, or fluid replacement.

B. Administer isotonic saline intravenously [incorrect]. Isotonic saline is a reasonable treatment provided that the patient is indeed hypovolemic.

C. Obtain laboratory tests to determine FE_{Na} [correct]. Basic laboratory tests and urine electrolytes will determine the volume status of the patient and how to proceed with volume augmentation as in choice B or administration of a diuretic.

D. Administer IV furosemide [incorrect]. Once volemic status has been determined, furosemide may be appropriate for euvolemic patients.

E. Administer dopamine [incorrect]. Dopamine can increase renal blood flow and glomerular filtration and therefore urine production.

15-A

A. Hepatitis B interferon [correct]. Membranous glomerulonephritis is the most common cause of nephrotic syndrome in adults. It is associated with hepatitis B; autoimmune disorders; and drugs such as gold salts, penicillamine, and captopril.

B. The amiodarone used for the treatment of her arrhythmia [incorrect]. Amiodarone, an antiarrhythmic used in the treatment of both ventricular and supraventricular arrhythmias, can cause hypothyroidism, corneal deposits, and interstitial lung disease, but is not classically associated with this renal disease.

C. The chemotherapy she receives for her Hodgkin lymphoma [incorrect]. Chemotherapy for Hodgkin lymphoma can include drugs such as bleomycin which is associated with interstitial lung disease.

D. The hydralazine she takes to control her blood pressure [incorrect]. Hydralazine is an antihypertensive that works by relaxing vascular smooth muscle. Its use has been associated with drug-induced lupus erythematosus.

E. The gentamicin she received while she was hospitalized for urosepsis [incorrect]. Gentamicin can cause nephrotoxicity as well as ototoxicity. The nephrotoxicity is usually defined as an increase in creatinine but can lead to severely impaired kidney function as a result of tubular damage.

16-E

A. Goodpasture syndrome [incorrect]. This disorder is caused by antibodies to the basement membrane proteins of the kidney and lung. Patients generally present with hemoptysis and hematuria.

B. Q fever [incorrect]. This type of pneumonia is caused by the zoonotic organism *Coxiella burnetii*. It is often transmitted to humans by livestock.

C. Osler-Weber-Rendu disease [incorrect]. This condition, also known as hereditary telangiectasia, presents with recurrent nose bleeds and/or GI bleeds along with telangiectatic skin lesions due to abnormal vascular proliferations.

D. Felty syndrome [incorrect]. RA, splenomegaly, and neutropenia compose the triad known as Felty syndrome. This condition has no significant pulmonary manifestations.

E. Kartagener syndrome [correct]. This condition is due to a defect in ciliary function and manifests with situs inversus, sinusitis, and bronchiectasis. The patient in this case has the classic findings of bronchiectasis.

17-C

A. Temozolomide [incorrect]. This is used in the treatment of glioblastoma multiforme. Indeed, glioblastoma multiforme can present as ring-enhancing masses; however, given the patient's HIV status, it is less likely.

B. Intrathecal methotrexate [incorrect]. Patients with primary CNS lymphoma can be treated with intrathecal methotrexate. Indeed, HIV patients are at increased risk but less likely in this scenario.

C. Pyrimethamine [correct]. *Toxoplasmosis gondii* is a parasitic organism acquired by exposure to cat feces or raw meat. It is much more common in HIV patients and is treated with pyrimethamine.

D. Dapsone and rifampin [incorrect]. Together these drugs are used to treat leprosy caused by the bacteria *Mycobacterium leprae*, which is exceedingly rare in the United States.

E. Intrathecal vancomycin [incorrect]. This drug can be used to treat bacterial meningitis as well as brain abscesses. Brain abscess can present as ring-enhancing masses on CT but are often more numerous.

18-E

A. Polymyalgia rheumatica [incorrect]. Polymyalgia rheumatica is an inflammatory condition primarily affecting those older than 70 years of age that presents with aches in the shoulder, hips, and proximal extremities.

B. Kawasaki disease [incorrect]. This disease involves the coronary arteries with the development of potential fatal aneurysmal dilation of such vessels. Children present with fever, a palmar rash, and a strawberry-colored tongue.

C. Behçet disease [incorrect]. This idiopathic autoinflammatory disease affects young adults and presents with recurrent aphthous ulcers, genital ulcers, and anterior uveitis.

D. Sjögren syndrome [incorrect]. This autoimmune disease involves the exocrine glands –and presents with parotid swelling, dry mouth, and dry eyes.

E. Takayasu arteritis [correct] An inflammatory involving the vessels of the aorta, Takayasu's disease (also known as pulseless disease), involves predominately young Asian women. It is managed with steroids or other immunodeficiency drugs.

19-B

A. Begin high-dose steroids [incorrect]. Indeed, corticosteroids may be indicated for this patient's case of silicosis; however, it would be prudent to complete the patient's workup as below.

B. Place a PPD [correct]. Patients with silicosis are at increased risk for the development of TB (silicotuberculosis). A PPD could help determine if this is the case in this patient. One would not want to give steroids to a patient with active TB.

C. Administer epinephrine [incorrect]. Epinephrine is the treatment for status asthmaticus. Because silicosis is a fibrotic disease, it is unlikely to provide much benefit in this patient.

D. Obtain a pleural biopsy [incorrect]. A pleural biopsy may be warranted to help evaluate for malignant mesothelioma. However, this tumor of the pleura is associated with asbestos exposure rather than silica exposure.

E. Treat the patient for allergic bronchopulmonary aspergillosis [incorrect]. This allergic disease is associated with *Aspergillus fumigatus*. It is treated with steroids, bronchodilators, and itraconazole.

20-E

A. It can be directly spread between infected persons [incorrect]. *Francisella tularensis*, like most zoonotic organisms, cannot be transmitted between humans.

B. A vaccine is available to the public [incorrect]. Although there are vaccines for other potential bioterrorism organisms such as anthrax and smallpox, no vaccine is available for *Francisella tularensis*.

C. The lethality results from the pneumonic and typhoidal forms of the diseases [incorrect]. In the era before antibiotics, mortality for the pneumonic and typhoidal forms of the disease approached 50%. This would make it a potent agent of bioterrorism, if it were not for antibiotics.

D. Infection is associated with infected cattle [incorrect]. Although infections such as brucellosis and anthrax are associated with cattle, tularemia is associated with infected rabbit hides.

E. The drug of choice for the treatment is streptomycin [correct]. Streptomycin is the antibiotic used to treat many of the zoonotic infections and is the drug of choice for the treatment of tularemia.

credits

Anatomical Chart Co. Fig. (54-1).

Armitage JO, Antman KH. *High-Dose Cancer Therapy: Pharmacology, Hematopoietins, Stem Cells.* 3rd ed. Philadelphia, PA: Lippincott Williams & Wilkins. Fig. 14, Ch. 35 (25-2).

Avner ED, Harmon WE, Niaudet P. *Pediatric Nephrology.* 5th ed. Philadelphia, PA: Lippincott Williams & Wilkins, 2003. Fig. 24.17 (48-1).

Bailey BJ, Johnson JT, et al. *Head and Neck Surgery—Otolaryngology.* 4th ed. Philadelphia, PA: Lippincott Williams & Wilkins, 2006. Fig. 46.1 (58-1); Table 25.2 (1-1).

Bhushan V, Le T, Pall V. *Underground Clinical Vignettes: Step 2 Internal Medicine II.* 3rd ed. Malden, MA: Blackwell Publishing, 2005. Figs. 10A (18-1), 10B (18-2), 10C (18-3), 20 (28-1), 23A (31-1), 23B (31-2), 27A (35-1), 27B (35-2), 39A (39-1), 39B (39-2), 36A (50-1), 36B (50-2), 45A (60-1), 45B (60-2), 46A (62-1), 46B (62-2), 48A (64-1), 48B (64-2), 51 (68-1), 53A (73-1), 53B (73-2), 53C (73-3).

Cagle PT. *Color Atlas & Text of Pulmonary Pathology.* Philadelphia, PA: Lippincott Williams & Wilkins, 2005. Fig. 10.42 (17-2).

Corman ML. *Colon & Rectal Surgery.* 5th ed. Philadelphia, PA: Lippincott Williams & Wilkins, 2004. Fig. 20-2 (14.1).

Crapo JD, Glassroth J, Karlinsky JB, King TE. *Baum's Textbook of Pulmonary Diseases.* 7th ed. Philadelphia, PA: Lippincott Williams & Wilkins, 2004. Figs. 27.5 (19-1), 62.5 (57-1), 44.9 (63-1).

DeLisa JA, Gans BM, et al. *Physical Medicine and Rehabilitation: Principles and Practice.* 4th ed. Philadelphia: Lippincott Williams & Wilkins, PA, 2004. Fig. 8-41 (66-1).

DeVita VT, Hellman S, Rosenberg SA. **Cancer:** *Principles and Practice of Oncology.* Philadelphia, PA: Lippincott Williams & Wilkins, 2004. Fig. 48.1-1 (14-2).

Eisenberg RL. *Clinical Imaging: An Atlas of Differential Diagnosis.* 4th ed. Philadelphia, PA: Lippincott Williams & Wilkins, 2002. Fig. B 10-11 (70-1).

Elder DE, Elenitsas R, et al. *Lever's Histopathology of the Skin.* 9th ed. Philadelphia, PA: Lippincott Williams & Wilkins, 2004. Figs. 20-1 (13-1), 20-2 (13-2), 9-6 (16-1).

Fleisher GR, Ludwig S, Baskin MN, eds. *Atlas of Pediatric Emergency Medicine.* Philadelphia, PA: Lippincott Williams & Wilkins, 2004. Fig. 11.2 (30-1).

Gillenwater JY, Grayhack JT, et al. *Adult and Pediatric Urology.* 4th ed. Philadelphia, PA: Lippincott Williams & Wilkins, 2001. Fig. 9.28A (47-1).

Gold DH, Weingeist TA. *Color Atlas of the Eye in Systemic Disease.* Baltimore, MD: Lippincott Williams & Wilkins, 2001. Fig. 15.2 (75-2).

Goodheart HP. *Goodheart's Photoguide of Common Skin Disorders.* 2nd ed. Philadelphia, PA: Lippincott Williams & Wilkins, 2003. Figs. 2.47 (11-1), 22.10 (17-1).

Gorbach SL, Bartlett JG, Blacklow NR. *Infectious Diseases.* 3rd ed. Philadelphia, PA: Lippincott Williams & Wilkins, 2003. Figs. 117.2 (26-1), 270.1 (27-1), 270.5 (27-2).

Greenspan A. *Orthopedic Imaging: A Practical Approach.* 4th ed. Philadelphia, PA: Lippincott Williams & Wilkins, 2004. Figs. 13.17 (67-1), 15.7 (72-1).

Hall JC. *Sauer's Manual of Skin Disorders.* 9th ed. Philadelphia, PA: Lippincott Williams & Wilkins, 2006. Fig. 22-4E (33-1).

Humes HD. *Kelley's Textbook of Internal Medicine.* 2nd ed. Philadelphia, PA: Lippincott Williams & Wilkins, 2001. Figs. 280.3 (24-1), 150.2A (43-1), 271.1 (51-1).

Keyes DC, Burstein JL, et al. *Medical Response to Terrorism: Preparedness and Clinical Practice.* Philadelphia, PA: Lippincott Williams & Wilkins, 2004. Fig. 11-6 (20-1).

Knipe DM, et al. *Field's Virology.* 5th ed. Philadelphia, PA: Lippincott Williams & Wilkins, 2006. Fig. 67.24 (25.1).

Lee JK, Sagel SS, et al. *Computed Body Tomography with MRI Correlation.* 4th ed. Philadelphia, PA: Lippincott Williams & Wilkins, 2005. Figs. 7-90 (55-1), 7-184 (63-2), 6-174 (75-1).

McClatchey KD, et al. *Clinical Laboratory Medicine.* 2nd ed. Philadelphia, PA: Lippincott Williams & Wilkins, 2001. Figs. 52.12 (22-1), 53.7 (23-1).

McMillan JA, Fergin RD, et al. *Oski's Pediatrics: Principles and Practice.* 4th ed. Philadelphia, PA: Lippincott Williams & Wilkins, 2006. Fig. 211.1 (22-2).

Oldham KT, Colombani PM, et al. *Principles and Practice of Pediatric Surgery.* Philadelphia, PA: Lippincott Williams & Wilkins, 2004. Fig. 55-8 (3-1).

Rubin E, Farber JL. *Pathology.* 3rd ed. Philadelphia, PA: Lippincott Williams & Wilkins, 1999. Figs. 24-72b (10-3), 24-26a (12-1).

Sauer GC. *Manual of Skin Diseases.* 5th ed. Philadelphia, PA: JB Lippincott, 1985. Fig. 44 (10-1).

Schrier RW. *Diseases of the Kidney and Urinary Tract.* 8th ed. Philadelphia, PA: Lippincott Williams & Wilkins, 2006. Fig. 15-4B (42-1).

Schwartz GR, Hanke BK, et al. *Principles and Practice of Emergency Medicine.* 4th ed. Philadelphia, PA: Lippincott Williams & Wilkins. Figs. 59-1.1 (5-1), 20-2.4 (60-3), 102-2.2 (65-1).

Shils ME, et al. *Modern Nutrition in Health and Disease.* 10th ed. Philadelphia, PA: Lippincott Williams & Wilkins, 2005. Fig. 95.1 (7-1).

Wachter RM, Goldman L, Hollander H. *Hospital Medicine.* 2nd ed. Philadelphia, PA: Lippincott Williams & Wilkins, 2005. Figs. 99.1b (41-1), 105.2 (49-1).

Wagner GS. *Marriott's Practical Electrocardiography.* 10th ed. Philadelphia, PA: Lippincott Williams & Wilkins, 2000. Figs. 11.17 (44-1), 11.9 (61-1).

Wolfson AB, et al. *Harwood-Nuss' Clinical Practice of Emergency Medicine.* 4th ed. Philadelphia, PA: Lippincott Williams & Wilkins, 2005. Table 132.1 (2-1).

case list

ALLERGY AND IMMUNOLOGY

1. Allergic Rhinitis
2. Angioedema
3. Aspirin-sensitive Asthma
4. Chronic Urticaria
5. Hymenoptera Hypersensitivity
6. Mastocytosis
7. Peanut Allergy
8. Penicillin Allergy
9. Severe Combined Immunodeficiency

DERMATOLOGY

10. Actinic Keratosis
11. Contact Dermatitis
12. Dermatitis Herpetiformis
13. Erythema Nodosum
14. Kaposi's Sarcoma
15. Psoriasis
16. Seborrheic Dermatitis
17. Squamous Cell Carcinoma

INFECTIOUS DISEASE

18. Amebic Liver Abscess
19. Aspergillosis: Allergic
20. Botulism
21. Cytomegalovirus Retinitis
22. Coccidioidomycosis
23. Epidemic Typhus
24. Gonorrhea
25. Herpes Genitalis
26. Herpes Zoster (Shingles)
27. Histoplasmosis
28. Infectious Mononucleosis
29. Legionella Pneumonia
30. Meningococcemia
31. Pneumococcal Pneumonia
32. Rubella (German Measles)
33. Syphilis: Secondary
34. Neurosyphilis (Tabes Dorsalis)
35. Tuberculosis: Pulmonary
36. Typhoid Fever
37. Cysticercosis
38. Meningitis: Cryptococcal
39. Septic Arthritis: Staphylococcal

NEPHROLOGY/UROLOGY

40. Acute Tubular Necrosis: Ischemic
41. Acute Tubular Necrosis: Toxic
42. Diabetic Nephropathy
43. Goodpasture Syndrome
44. Hyperkalemia
45. Membranous Glomerulonephritis
46. Minimal-Change Disease
47. Nephrolithiasis
48. Postinfectious Glomerulonephritis
49. Renal Tubular Acidosis
50. Renovascular Hypertension: Fibromuscular Dysplasia
51. Urinary Tract Infection

PULMONARY

52. Adult Respiratory Distress Syndrome
53. Asbestosis
54. Asthma: Chronic
55. Chronic Obstructive Pulmonary Disease: Chronic Bronchitis
56. Chronic Obstructive Pulmonary Disease: Emphysema
57. Marfan Syndrome
58. Obstructive Sleep Apnea
59. Pleural Effusion

index